S0-AIT-130

MALE
MULTIPLE
ORGASM

MALE MULTIPLE ORGASM

TECHNIQUES THAT GUARANTEE YOU AND YOUR LOVER INTENSE SEXUAL PLEASURE **AGAIN** AND **AGAIN** AND **AGAIN**

SOMRAJ POKRAS

Amorata Press

Text Copyright © 2007 Somraj Pokras. Design Copyright © 2007 Ulysses Press and its licensors. All rights reserved under International and Pan-American Copyright Conventions, including the right to reproduce this book or portions thereof in any form whatsoever, except for use by a reviewer in connection with a review.

Published by: AMORATA PRESS,
an imprint of Ulysses Press
P.O. Box 3440
Berkeley, CA 94703
www.amoratapress.com

ISBN10: 1-56975-625-2
ISBN13: 978-1-56975-625-6
Library of Congress Control Number: 2007906079

Printed in the United States by Bang Printing

10 9 8 7 6 5 4 3 2 1

Acquisitions Editor: Nick Denton-Brown
Managing Editor: Claire Chun
Editor: Joanna Pearlman
Editorial and production staff: Judith Metzener, Emma Silvers, Elyce Petker
Cover design: what!design @ whatweb.com
Cover photo: ©iStockphoto.com/g_studio

Distributed by Publishers Group West

This book has been written and published strictly for informational purposes, and in no way should it be used as a substitute for consultation with professional therapists. All facts in this book came from scientific publications, personal interviews, published trade books, self-published materials by experts, magazine articles, and the personal-practice experiences of the authorities quoted or sources cited. The author and publisher are providing you with information in this work so that you can have the knowledge and can choose, at your own risk, to act on that knowledge.

I dedicate this book to my lovely and accomplished wife,
Dr. Jeffre TallTrees,
who supported me while I struggled to learn to celebrate life
as well as she does, and who both helped me in this process
and benefited tremendously from learning to make love for hours.

✧ Contents

✧ *Introduction*

My name is Somraj, and I'm a retired corporate trainer turned sex researcher. As long as I can remember, I've been a horny guy. I was never good at overcoming premature ejaculation because nobody taught me how to make sex last longer.

I've always thought of myself as a real man—you know, a macho guy. But I've always been real sensitive, too. Yes, I'm referring to having a hair trigger that made me come too quickly during sex, which didn't do a lot for my virile self-image. Neither did my inability to give my then (now ex-) wife an orgasm during intercourse.

Like any modern man, I never avoided any challenge that tempted me. So when I met a circle of guys who could last as long as they wanted to in bed, I decided to do something about my situation. *Male Multiple Orgasm* is my story about how I learned to...

Have multiple orgasms,

Make love for hours and enjoy it more,

Enjoy all sorts of bigger and better orgasms, and

Develop unlimited sexual stamina.

When I started this personal quest, I didn't plan to write this story or share it with anybody. I just wasn't feeling good about myself and needed some help. So I reached out and found out that, lo and behold, there was a lot I didn't know about sex, lovemaking, and, especially, premature ejaculation. Duh!

I discovered that the answers are out there, they're just scattered and hidden. Some techniques are the result of the modern science they call "sexology." But most of the techniques have been around for thousands of years. I experimented with everything I came across until I figured out what worked best. Amazingly, with lots of practice, I learned how to enjoy sex without ejaculating before I wanted.

That's when I decided to collect all these workable longer-sex secrets together in one place. Since my career had been writing training manuals and conducting people-skills workshops for Fortune 500 firms, I naturally chose to write a how-to guide. That's why the most important elements of *Male Multiple Orgasm* are its simple step-by-step exercises.

Because this book is all about strengthening sexual muscles and developing sexual skills, the exercises it contains are natural, permanent, and without side effects. Well, unless you call being urged to go to bed more often a side effect.

Many of the practices that are going to revolutionize your sexual stamina and orgasms are based on modern techniques. But the best, the most powerful, the most natural, and truly the core methods come from Tantra, often called sacred sexuality. So I want to explain just a bit what Tantra is all about.

The friends who started me on this journey were adept in the ancient Eastern spiritual practice called Tantra. Thousands of years ago, the original mystics developed methods of working with the energy in the body that made people feel better, stay healthier, and be more conscious. Since sex is probably the strongest source of physical energy, the ancient Tantrikas used it to gain mastery over pleasure, orgasm, and bliss. When the Tantrikas eventually were persecuted, Tantra went underground until some adventuresome teachers resurrected it in the modern West.

Thanks to these teachers and friends who helped me overcome premature ejaculation, now you, too, can learn Male Multiple Orgasm techniques. Lasting longer is very possible to learn, if you want to. You simply need to reprogram yourself and develop some new skills. If you're interested enough to read this book and spend some time changing your love life, then we're not so different, you and me. So I'm confident, with a little dedication, time, and regular practice, this method will work for you. I know, because of the men and their lovers that I've helped through our website, TantraAtTahoe.com, since the late 1990s.

Frankly, reprogramming your body, mind, and spirit probably won't happen instantly. This is why I make such a big deal about practicing. That's where your transformation will really happen. But the good news is that, whether you get the knack fast or slow, you'll be practicing something that feels really good and yields clear-cut results.

If it helps you carry on, just ask yourself this: "Would you like to be able to look any woman in the eye and know with total confidence that you could satisfy her beyond her wildest dreams?" That's what kept me going, getting me to this place where I can say to myself with certainty, "Yes, I would."

As you're getting there, I'd love to hear about your progress with the exercises in *Male Multiple Orgasm* via email through my website, TantraAtTahoe.com.

Best of luck and enjoy.

Somraj Pokras
Truckee, California
September 2007

CHAPTER 1

✧ *Welcome to Orgasm Mastery*

This book is about how to become an Orgasm Master, about how to enjoy lots more sexual pleasure for an extended period of time. Additionally, you're going to learn to voluntarily have different "kinds" of orgasms than you're used to, as many as you want for as long as you choose. By reading *Male Multiple Orgasm*, you're jumping on a train whose destination is continuous ecstatic feelings far better than any quick flash in the pan. Now doesn't that sound like mastery?

You're going to discover (if you don't already know) that ejaculation doesn't always have to accompany orgasm. That's how those who've learned the techniques in this book have multiple orgasms, spasm after spasm, that seem to go on forever— but without the wet release that, for most of us, ends the fun.

As an Orgasm Master, you'll be able to choose when you want to ejaculate. After some months of extended practice, when you're having so many dry orgasms that feel so incredible, you may decide to have fewer wet ones. Or none at all. It's OK if you're thinking, "No way, I enjoy it too much." I'm not going to argue with that desire, since that's how most men feel. Since you'll be the master, you can choose to do what gives you the most pleasure.

Just let me ask you this: "What will you choose if you learn to transform the sexual energy of your orgasms into an unlimited current of sensation that feels so much better and reaches so much higher than a few seconds of release?"

THE CURE FOR INVOLUNTARY EJACULATION

Contrary to what you might have heard from guys who tell you to think about baseball or your grandmother to keep from orgasming, *Male Multiple Orgasm* is about MORE ecstasy, not LESS. The experts say that sexual response has four stages: excitation, plateau, orgasm, and resolution. The last stage is where your body goes back to normal. The aim here is simply to lengthen the plateau phase indefinitely. That's why this book is about Orgasm Mastery, not about control. Control implies staying under tension, always being careful, and not trusting yourself to relax. That's the opposite of the direction we're moving here.

Mastery Means Separating Orgasm from Ejaculation

Let me give you a taste of what's to come. Here's an excerpt from an erotic story I wrote about an actual experience:

"I thrust slowly, to appreciate every millimeter of sensation, intense with pleasure. I wanted to savor each sensation fully. She was rocking and moaning with pleasure, making me want to come. I breathed, relaxed, and circulated the sensations up and away from my genitals, into the other parts of my body. The intense urge to ejaculate calmed and I relaxed into more intense stimulation. By circulating the sensation out of my genitals and into the other parts of my body, it felt like I was coming all over in little orgasmic explosions. These spasms that spread all over were so delightful that I just let them run their course. Each little stroke was ecstatic all by itself, creating intense feelings of pleasure. The pleasure from each movement was so overpowering that I could have stopped after any one of them and felt as sexually complete as if I'd just ejaculated. Instead, I continued making love, making her shake with ecstasy, as we rose over and over to just before the point of no return."

Who would want all this pleasure to end quickly in just a few seconds of explosion instead?

Inherent in separating orgasm from ejaculation is that you will be able to time your explosion to experience a wet orgasm at the moment you choose. This offers hope to the millions of men who feel that they let loose too quickly. If you are one of these men, ejaculating quickly doesn't mean that you're broken. In fact, it's more common than you might think. It's just not the kind of thing most guys want to discuss over a cold one.

I've come to realize that there's nothing physically wrong with us sensitive types. Being quick on the draw is basically the product of how we've been taught—or not taught—and conditioned about sex. You know, like trying to release all that tension with your hand. Or to get your first romps on the couch or backseat over with before you get caught. Face it, guy, this is how we learned to have sex! So all I'm hoping to do in *Male Multiple Orgasm* is show you a new pattern to practice.

Only 2 Minutes?

According to some estimates, about 30% of American men reach orgasm earlier than they'd like. Alfred Kinsey, one of the earliest and best-known American sex researchers, found that 75% of the men he tested ejaculated within two minutes of vaginal entry.

So if you think you orgasm too quickly, you're not alone. And it's nothing to be ashamed of. Orgasming is a good thing; it just may not always happen when you want it to. Consider it a timing problem that, in the overwhelming majority of cases, is easily corrected with training. Researchers have shown that involuntary orgasm is not a physical disability and that it is nearly 95% curable. You simply need to spend some time reprogramming yourself and developing some new skills.

There is a very small chance, however, that you have a medical condition causing your timing problem. It's a good idea to have a doctor check out your equipment if you suspect anything less than robust health "down there."

What Women Really Want

In addition to teaching you to enjoy endless sexual ecstasy, *Male Multiple Orgasm* will teach you the techniques you need to become the best, most sensitive, longest-lasting lover you can be. These are the skills that will help you drive your woman wild in bed, bringing her to new heights of sexual pleasure.

But be aware that different women like different things. Many women have their own personal issues, which block them from reaching full sexual ecstasy no matter how skilled their lovers may be.

My previous wife didn't have vaginal orgasms, no matter what we did. I felt that it was my failure, but in retrospect, I did everything I could to pleasure her. In reality, it wasn't my fault.

Many women (some studies indicate up to 75%) don't have orgasms through intercourse. So, if you're driving yourself crazy trying to do the impossible with a particular woman, lighten up!

I'm not trying to talk you out of learning the skills in this book to better enjoy sex. I'm just trying to inject a little reality. If you learn to make love for hours, some women will really, really love it. But some may not. And some may never have the kind of explosion most guys seem to crave. You'll have to accept the limitations of your individual situation.

That being said, with *Male Multiple Orgasm* you will absolutely become a much better lover, capable of sustaining the ultimate in sexual pleasure for as long as you choose.

TANTRA AND TANTRIC SEX

Many techniques that can help you become multi-orgasmic have their roots in ancient sources like Tantra, an ancient Eastern spiritual practice based on the metaphysics of sexual energy. Tantra can teach you how to harness the forces inside you that drive sex to improve your body, mind, and spirit. So Tantra is often called spiritual sex or sacred sexuality.

Tantra's roots are very old. It emerged thousands of years ago in India in secret writings that described sexual rituals, disciplines, and meditations as a path toward personal enlightenment. Tantra shows you how to accept and love all that you are so you can open fully to your sexual and spiritual nature. That, the story goes, allows you to experience more pleasure and more ecstasy for longer times.

Tantric Sex Is Subtle Energy Exchange

Tantra teaches that all energy, including the incredible power in your orgasms, is a vital part of who you are. When you're learn-

---

TANTRIC WRITINGS

The earliest Tantras—secret writings—exalted the cult of the god Shiva, one of the primary Hindu deities, and his consort, the goddess Shakti. Hindus believed that Shakti created the universe by uniting spiritually and sexually with Shiva. This erotic love creation-myth certainly builds different core values than the Adam and Eve story that most of us learned as kids. Here is just one example of Tantra's pragmatic, non-dogmatic, approach to living. We borrow myths, principles, and rituals from other disciplines that help our inner beings grow. But we don't use them to judge, grade, or police our behavior.

Today, Tantrikas revere Shiva as the pure embodiment of the masculine force culminating in cosmic consciousness, and Shakti as the feminine principle embodying pure creative energy. This isn't worship of supreme beings as in other religions. Rather, it's our way of honoring the forces of nature that exist within all of us. We simply use Shiva and Shakti as convenient symbols to focus the growth of our own divine qualities. In short, Tantrikas honor our inner male and female, regardless of our biological gender.

ing to tap into this reservoir of life force, it seems subtle, like trying to hear a sound with a frequency much higher than you're used to hearing. You'll find this power sometimes referred to as sexual energy or its strongest incarnation, orgasmic energy.

Tantra uses orgasmic energy practices to...

- Deepen your love, intimacy and ecstasy,
- Extend your sexual stamina and lengthen your lovemaking, and
- Create continuous earth-shattering orgasms.

Maybe Tantra has been around so long because of the huge inner reservoirs of untapped power you can access using its practices. Or maybe it's just because of the amazing ecstasy you can generate by making love in this unique way, which we call Tantric Sex.

For all these reasons, my definition of the kind of sex you'll be learning here is S.E.X., which stands for Subtle Energy eXchange.

What Will It Take to Change Your Sex Life Forever?

Tantra can help you become the confident, satisfied, playful, energetic lover you were born to be, a lover who has the desire and capacity for making loveplay last through multiple orgasms of multiple kinds.

You might have heard that *Tantrikas* (practitioners adept at Tantra) and other Eastern gurus give up ejaculation entirely or become celibate. If you're worried about what you're getting yourself into, don't be. Tantra isn't a religion based on faith, dogma, or right living. You don't have to join a movement, carry a card, cut your hair, or wear robes. I just want you to know where the unique essence of *Male Multiple Orgasm* comes from.

My wife and I have been teaching men and their lovers how to use orgasmic energy this way since the 1990s. In large part, our actual experience using the essence of the ancient Tantric teachings is where this book came from. Also, I've researched and added methods from modern psychology and sexology, bringing you the best of the old world and the new.

In Chapter 3, I'll explain the heart and soul of that unique essence, the six-step formula that's going to, with your cooperation, change your sex life forever.

But first, in Chapter 2, we'll do a brief review of male sexual anatomy and the physical experience of a male erection.

CHAPTER 2

✧ *The Mechanics*
of Male Sex

Before we get started with the practices that will make you an Orgasm Master, we need to look briefly into what happens inside when guys experience sex. In this chapter, we'll review male sexual anatomy, the two stages of ejaculation, what causes it to happen before you want, and how you're going to change all that.

MALE SEXUAL ANATOMY

It's a good bet that you're familiar with the overall experience of ejaculating. First you get turned on, and then you feel so excited you can't control it, and finally you have to let go. You ejaculate, and then get soft. But there's more to it than that.

I'm talking about the very pleasurable ten-second involuntary muscle contractions that we call male orgasm. Sometimes the contractions start mild and get stronger, but once you pass the point of no return with that first spasm, releasing semen to the outside world is inevitable for most of us. Believe it or not, you're going to learn to make those involuntary muscle contractions respond to your power of choice.

We're all aware of the obvious outcome of an explosive orgasm that I just described. To be an Orgasm Master, you need to become much more aware of the internal process leading up to explosive climax, as well as the anatomy behind it. Then you'll be in a position to change the sequence of events that leads to losing it.

To learn to separate ejaculation from orgasm when you want to, it helps to be familiar with the entire sexual territory "down there." How can you become an expert if you don't know all the parts?

A Penis by Any Other Name

If you're a male, I know you're already intimately familiar with your pleasure stick. Since we're just regular guys talking here (right?), I won't be using the term "penis" much. I prefer the spiritual view, that your male member is a divine gift designed largely for your pleasure. With this mindset, a clinical approach doesn't fit. So I'm going to use the Tantric term *vajra*, which literally means "divine thunderbolt" in Sanskrit.

Whatever you call it, vajra is a great tool to have hanging around, don't you agree?

Vajra is a highly sensitive, expandable, male organ that so many of us, whatever our gender, love to play with. As you can see from Figure 1, his head and tip are technically called the *glans*. (If you're an uncircumcised male, your foreskin usually covers the glans.) The glans is pretty darn sensi-

tive, as is the crest around it, known as the *corona or coronal ridge*. Most guys report that the *frenulum*, the soft area on vajra's underside below the corona, is the most sensitive.

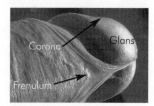

Figure 1: Circumcised penis

You know vajra swells when excited, right? But do you know how?

In spite of such slang names as "boner" and "woody," there are no bones or tree trunks inside vajra. He contains spongy erectile tissue that expands when blood flows in, part of which is shown in Figure 2. Isn't it wonderful that he gets big and hard when he fills with blood that stays put? That's where erections, or hard-ons, come from.

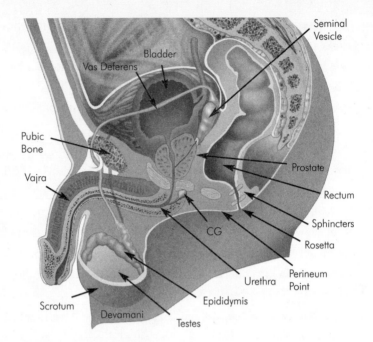

Figure 2: Male Sexual Anatomy

Vajra's Got Some Pretty Spiffy Neighbors

Did you get an owner's manual when you were issued your jewels, my preferred term for genitals? I guess not. What hangs out between your legs may be obvious, but not all your sexual anatomy is external. Let's dig into Figure 2, starting at the manufacturing end of your production line, and trace your sexual geography from one end to the other to make sure you understand all your equipment.

Did you ever hear the joke that uses another name for vajra, the one with the punch line "Big Jim and the Twins"? I've never met a guy who didn't laugh when calling his member Big Jim. The twins, of course, are those two balls that hang beneath vajra.

Officially, Big Jim's neighbors are called *testes* or testicles. These two egg-shaped glands ride in your *scrotum*, the sac made from folds of skin. The testes glands are where your sperm cells are manufactured. They also secrete *testosterone*, the hormone that drives the sex lives of both men and women.

To get away from all the dirty jokes and unwanted connotations, I prefer the Sanskrit term *devamani* (divine jewels) for Big Jim's twins.

Since we're being picky here, you might as well learn about the *epididymis*, the storage area for new sperm that's wrapped around the upper end of each devamani. These brave little swimmers grow and mature in these special bags until they're strong enough for travel and competition.

When you let go, their route is up the two *spermatic ducts* called the *vas* or *ductus deferens*. These firm, muscular tubes coil up and around your bladder and meet at your prostate gland. It's the two vas that get cut if you have a *vasectomy* (after which your sperm cells have nowhere to go). Though there are actually two of them—one from each devamani—that pass on either side of the bladder, you can only see the top in the cross-section view in Figure 2.

To the right of the bladder you can see the vas connecting with one of the two *seminal vesicles*, which are little sacs about the size of your small finger. This is where most of the fluid comes from when you ejaculate.

Your Prostate Gland

If you look carefully at Figure 2, under the bladder you can find your *prostate* gland. The prostate is egg-shaped or round and about the shape and size of a chestnut or walnut. It's half glandular and half muscular, which makes its fibrous mass feel much harder than the rest of the surrounding tissue.

Your gland secretes *prostatic fluid*, a colorless, odorless, slightly milky and salty, semi-viscous liquid that's a part of semen. Prostatic fluid often tastes sweet because it contains sugar as a nutrient for sperm. It also carries hormones that make fertilization more likely when a guy ejaculates inside a fertile woman's vagina.

Why is understanding this anatomy important? Because the prostate is where ejaculation begins, with the contractions of the muscle sheath around the gland. As you learn to become an Orgasm Master, you'll become well acquainted with this reflex.

You can see one of the (unlabeled) *ejaculatory ducts* running from the visible seminal vesicle through the prostate connected to the *urethra*. The *urethra* is a tube that runs from your bladder through the middle of your prostate to the end of vajra. The urethra conveys both urine and semen to the outside world, but fortunately not at the same time. So that urine can't leave the bladder during ejaculation, the prostate gland closes off the upper end of the urethra while vajra is employed in more pleasurable pursuits.

Right below the prostate you can see the yellow cross-sections of the pelvic muscles, which I call PC, short for pubococcygeus. You'll soon become expert in using these muscles to extend your sexual stamina.

Perineum Point: A Window Inside

Your *perineum* is the soft area at the base of your pelvic floor, midway between your devamani and *rosetta*, my preferred name for that rose-shaped orifice held tight by your round anal sphincter muscle.

Why is this spot between your balls and anus in Figure 2 labeled *perineum point*?

If you press inward and upward on your perineum when vajra is soft, you'll feel your pelvic bone close to your scrotum and a soft spongy area closer to rosetta. That's your perineum point, important because, under the arrowhead, you can massage your prostate from the outside.

If you explore when vajra is hard, ahead of your perineum you'll probably feel vajra's root or bulb. That's the inside end of your erection, not shown in Figure 2. Like so much of the territory we've explored here, your perineum point will come in handy later on as you learn to master your orgasms.

Sweet Dribblings Are Nothing to Worry About

Our journey is almost done after this one last vital stop. The *Cowper's Glands* are just a bit downstream from the prostate. They're labeled "CG" in the drawing. Just before release, they emit a clear, colorless, thickish, alkaline liquid that helps to lubricate the canal sperm travel through. This *preejaculate* also neutralizes any acidic remains of urine in the urethra. Got to keep those little swimmers as happy as possible until the very last moment.

I get quite a few emails from guys who are worried if their vajras drip after practicing this program. I'm officially telling you now: DON'T WORRY.

This dripping from the end of vajra after lots of play without ejaculation is likely your unannounced meeting with the Cowper's product. Actually, it's good news, being part of nature's plan to lubricate vajra's head. So, if you find as you work through the program in this book that you're dribbling more than you used to, don't worry about it. It just means you're spending more time turned on than before.

By the way, if the fluid is colored, seeps in great volume, or leaks without prostate stimulation, you should see a doctor to check it out.

But there is some other news about preejaculate that you should be aware of. It can transport the remaining sperm cells hanging around from previous sexual escapades. That's why intercourse with early withdrawal or without ejaculation isn't a reliable birth control method.

EJACULATION STAGES

Though that's the end of the anatomy lesson, we're going to walk through the process of ejaculation. You're undoubtedly aware of the signs that you're about to have an orgasm. Your skin gets flushed. Your breathing speeds up to the point of panting. Your heart rate and blood pressure rapidly increase. Your legs and butt tense. Your pelvic muscles tighten up.

What may not be as obvious is that your devamani elevate and draw up against your body, vajra swells, and your prostate fills with fluid in preparation for ejaculation. This sets you up for making a big wet spot.

Right before you lose it and become oblivious to the outside world for a while, time stops and you feel yourself teetering on the edge of the cliff. That's because the initial release is usually involuntary and outside an untrained man's level of consciousness. You're going to change that by getting intimately familiar with this moment of ejaculatory inevitability that I so affectionately call *the point of no return*.

A Two-Stage Process

Did you know that going over the side with a wet explosion is really a two-stage process? It is. There's emission and expulsion.

During the emission phase, the two long vas deferens tubes contract and propel sperm up from their storage areas, the epididymis, in your devamani. Your sperm cells pass through the ejaculatory ducts in your prostate as its muscular sheath contracts, mixing with fluid from the prostate, seminal vesicles, and Cowper's Glands. All these seminal fluids get emptied into your urethra, mixing together to form semen.

Then the expulsion phase takes over, and rhythmic, wavelike PC muscle contractions propel semen down the urethra and out vajra's head, where those little swimmers have a brief fight for survival. They usually lose, except for the rare one that finds its way to fertilize an egg (technically an *ovum*, a female reproductive cell), resulting in pregnancy.

Scientists who study orgasms tell us that the average guy is likely to have 10 to 15 spasms that last a little less than a second each. It's the contractions of the PC pelvic muscles that cause the actual release of semen. Plus, they're the main source of pleasure during orgasm.

How You'll Learn Male Multiple Orgasm

Here's what's in store for you: You're going to make **voluntary** what's normally **involuntary**, at least where it comes to sexual discharge. In other words, you're going to be able to time orgasms and choose when to ejaculate. By strengthening your PC muscles, learning to relax, and heightening your awareness of the whole process, you'll learn to avoid the emission stage altogether.

But remember, it's the PC contractions of the expulsion that feel so good. You'll still get to enjoy the wonderful orgasmic ecstasy of those spasms without making a wet spot. Most guys I know call these "dry orgasms."

The best news of all: After a dry orgasm, vajra can get less sensitive for a while, so you can pump vigorously again. And there's no reason why you can't repeat this entire cycle as many times as you want.

That is, when you want to have Male Multiple Orgasms.

There's an even better way to describe how you're going to learn to time your wet explosions. Most guys build up sexual tension through more and more arousal until they seemingly have no other option but to release the sexual energy by ejaculating.

The Male Multiple Orgasm method of mastering dry orgasms and unlimited sexual stamina means you will learn to recirculate the energy within your body. When you spread the excitement all over, not only does it feel great, but the urge to ejaculate subsides. You might say that sexual energy conservation is the real secret and the true power of Male Multiple Orgasm.

CAUSES OF PREMATURE EJACULATION

If it bums you out to think about all that goes wrong when you climax too soon, you might be tempted to skip this section. But don't. Though I'm sure you know some of the causes of premature ejaculation, I'll bet you aren't aware of all of the factors that can cause too-rapid timing of your orgasm. In fact, after a long career of ejaculatory mastery, some men lose it temporarily because one or more of the causes listed below rear their ugly heads.

The Urge to Ejaculate

I want to hit the biggie right on the head at the outset here. When we get turned on, something inside takes over and convinces us to just let go. There always used to be a rationalization in my head that seemed to make sense in the moment why I should go ahead and ejaculate. I usually regretted it later.

It may sound like circular reasoning to say that the urge to ejaculate is the reason you ejaculate too quickly. We all have the urge to orgasm, right? Well, of course. And I don't want to give you the idea that there's anything wrong with it. The craving for pleasure is what life is about. But what kind of orgasm are we talking about seeking here? Yours, a quickie, your lover's, or a full-body multiple one? The biological urge to ejaculate seems to circumvent your voluntary power of choice in the matter.

As a result of my more than 30 years' experience helping people change their behavior, I'm convinced that few succeed at STOPPING something they don't want to give up. The secret is to replace what you don't want with something better that you DO want. Fortunately, *Male Multiple Orgasm* offers something much better. Once you develop the knack of inner orgasm from practicing the exercises in this book, you'll never want to go back and spray your seed outside.

Overwhelming Excitement

This must have happened to all of us at least once. You're really attracted to that completely sexy thing who actually wants to have sex with you. You're so turned on by the whole prospect that before you know it, you ejaculate in your shorts or, even worse, all over her skirt.

God, I hate remembering those embarrassing times, and wouldn't mention premature ejaculation if I wasn't confident this will soon be a thing of the past for you.

Being overwhelmingly excited is part of being a red-blooded healthy male. The younger a man is, the more excitable he tends to be. It's common that the first few times young, inexperienced men have sex with a partner, they have trouble controlling their response. Since we haven't been taught any other way, we just blindly follow the natural flood surging inside us and soon our pants are wet. Many of us just haven't learned that there is another way to deal with the huge energy build-up.

If you're young, patient, and willing to wait a decade or three, high excitability may mellow with age. If you'd like a solution sooner, read on.

Tension & Anxiety

The secret to ejaculatory mastery is relaxation. There are so many things that can create tension and anxiety in the scary arena of sex, I'm actually astounded how many men learn to pace themselves in the sack. Here are just a few of the common stresses that can cause too-rapid ejaculation:

- time pressure
- self-doubt
- religious guilt, thinking sex is bad, dirty, or immoral
- fear of getting caught
- tiredness or sickness
- relationship stress
- worries about pregnancy or STDs (sexually transmitted diseases)
- performance anxiety ("Am I good enough to satisfy my partner?")
- trying not to ejaculate

Can you believe that last one? Thinking about not ejaculating can actually make you more likely to explode too soon. Amazing, but true.

Conditioning to Go Fast

Sex therapists claim that climaxing quickly begins during youth and then becomes an unconscious, physically ingrained habit that persists later in life. Haven't most of us grown up being afraid of getting discovered having sex? Remember, many of our first sexual encounters were rushing it in the back seat of our dad's Chevy or on the living room couch with the folks due back any minute. We were so worried about getting caught in the act that sex was often hurried and less than it could have been.

And what about making it with our first partner—our hand? To limit our chances of being found out, masturbating quickly for a fast release is the norm for most guys. To relieve the sexual tension, we just tried to get it over with in secret as rapidly as possible. When we had our first orgasms in the bathroom, while showering, or in bed, we were anxiously hoping we wouldn't get caught.

While our bodies are tense from being so horny, our minds end up under psychological tension as well. As a result, we get programmed to get sex over with quickly.

Goal of Orgasm

We live in a world structured around goals, standards, and living up to expectations. What's the media-driven performance standard for the ideal macho male lover? You should know women so well that you please any and all of them. You play each one so well until she loses control and her desire overpowers good sense and any inhibitions. Until she goes completely berserk with passion, you're the strong silent type. Then, in a wild release proving that you're the best, you and your lover have a monstrous orgasm simultaneously.

Face it, guys, the Big O (a strong explosive orgasm) is what our sexually repressed and unevolved society measures us against. We're raised with the belief that the purpose of making love is to release all that pent-up sexual energy with the most intense orgasm possible. Often, we get trapped in our partner's similar belief, driven by long periods of being unsatisfied sexually.

As wonderful as orgasm is, you might be surprised to learn how important many other things are (cuddling, caring, sensitivity) to the average woman. I read a study recently that quoted 70% of women would choose intimacy over sex.

We're programmed to rush headlong toward orgasm as fast as we can go. In our haste, we miss many sensations and experiences along the way. The Western view of sex is a race to the climax, after which lovers physically collapse. Except that few of the women I know want you to roll over and snore just then.

Male Multiple Orgasm is closer to the Eastern view of physical love, which slowly brings both partners to higher and higher heights of ecstasy time and time again. That's what we're aiming to master here.

The Mind

Without a doubt, the mind is a powerful sex organ. Many spiritual teachers have shown us that "where attention goes, energy flows." Focus on pleasure and your experience becomes more intense. Think about not ejaculating and you will do it anyway.

We all attract what we focus on. For example, if your whole attention is on your jewels, then your sexual energy has nowhere else to go but out that little hole in vajra's head. If you're intent on the goal of giving your partner an orgasm, then you're likely to attract one too soon—namely one of your own. Case histories of psychological reasons for premature ejaculation abound.

Male Multiple Orgasm is about learning to enjoy sex even more while managing ejaculation. The mind's tricks—goals or mental images that are totally absorbing—get in the way of you tuning into the present moment. With these consuming internal distractions, how can you truly appreciate what's happening now? Instead, you need to shift your attention into the now and onto your senses, whole body, feelings, and sensations. Focus on all the imaginable sources of pleasure. We'll discuss more about this later.

You might say the essence of *Male Multiple Orgasm* is to get out of your head and into your body. Relax and stay in the moment, tuning into those wonderful feelings emanating from your sensitive places. Drop all your standards and goals, and just ride the wave of energy. Don't push yourself or your partner for the Big O.

Here's your unlimited sexual stamina formula in a nutshell: When you learn to surf your sexual energy without attempting to control the outcome, you'll be able to go with the flow in a loose and natural way indefinitely.

Separate, Not Joint, Experience

In our society, for the most part, sex is a private experience because it's a taboo subject. We hide our insecurities, make rude jokes, and don't talk about what we're really feeling openly. Too many of us obsess about when to make the first move, or even about how to initiate with a long-time partner, instead of joyously enjoying verbal foreplay. No wonder so many of us build up the anxieties and tensions we talked about earlier that can cause premature ejaculation.

We're not taught that sex is communion between souls expressing their basic nature through the divine gift of bodies. Few of us learn to play these instruments in harmony to produce amazing ecstasy. Where do we learn that sex is an energy exchange between conscious beings who want to both give and receive pleasure?

When you're desired and accepted for who you are without big expectations about how you need to perform, then you can relax and let nature take its sexual course. That's partly why *Male Multiple Orgasm* requires "partnering" with your lover. This means being aware of your needs and reactions, talking honestly about them, honoring those of your partner, and playing together as equals. Instead of "doing" your partner, you'll need to do such things as sharing together.

By the way, everything in *Male Multiple Orgasm* is completely applicable to same gender sex. Tantra has a lot to say about yin and yang energies, which we normally associate with female and male genders. But experienced practitioners learn that we all have both energies within and can act on both if we practice. I've tried to make the language inoffensive to gay and lesbian partners, but I probably haven't done a perfect job. So please accept this disclaimer that everything included is applicable and intended for you, too. In fact, S.E.X. being Subtle Energy eXchange probably applies even more for same-sex partners.

Different partners have different sexual responses. Some women can reach orgasm very quickly, but most need lots of stimulation. Myself, I always like lots of touching all over my body. If vajra gets too much attention too quickly, the rest of me doesn't get turned on and it's all over for both of us too soon. So who's responsible for seeing that each partner gets the things that bring the most pleasure? We each are fully responsible. Partnering means speaking your needs and honoring those of your partner. If we do anything else, we set up the dynamics that produce stress, mystery, and tension—a surefire prescription for ejaculating unexpectedly.

If you're single and searching for a partner to satisfy sexually, this whole view of sex as communion may sound even more challenging than finding someone willing to jump in the sack. If you expect that you alone will be able to satisfy any woman without her cooperation, you're laboring under a big delusion, friend. Drop the whole concept that it's your job ALONE to satisfy your partner. This is a mutual dance and that's the way most women love it. Later, I'll show you how to broach this delicate subject with potential partners that will make you seem more desirable to them, not less.

Prostatitis

Being part of the first emission phase of ejaculation, the prostate gland is a vital component of your sexual equipment. If it's inflamed or enlarged, called *prostatitis*, it can easily make you more sensitive to stimulation and more likely to let go at a moment's notice. If you're very sensitive down there or have trouble peeing, get a referral from your physician to a urologist (a medical doctor who specializes in that part of your body). And if you're taking any prescription drugs, discuss possible sexual side effects with your doctor or pharmacist.

Fortunately, there are some natural remedies that can improve your prostate health. I take Saw Palmetto and Pygeum daily, two natural herbs you can get at the health food store. Research has shown these supplements can help your prostate significantly.

While we're on the subject, there are some other common substances that can inflame your prostate and make you more sensitive to premature ejaculation. Can you guess what they are? Right, I'm talking about caffeine, nicotine, and alcohol. If you smoke, drink caffeinated beverages such as coffee or cola, and/or drink alcohol, you would be well advised to avoid them during this program.

Believe me, I'm not a moralist trying to convince you of your evil ways. I've tried most everything and believe in whatever brings pleasure. When I'm warning you about irritating your prostate, it's just a medical fact. Alcohol and smoking are the primary reasons that men over age 30 have erection problems. Other medications and recreational drugs can have significant effects on your sexual mastery as well.

General Health

As I just explained, Male Multiple Orgasm will go better if you avoid any stimulants that inflame your prostate. It's a completely natural program that depends on your general health. So, eating well, taking care of yourself, and staying in shape will help. Then you'll have the stamina to exercise longer and harder both in and out of bed.

Also, sex requires physical energy, which is drawn from your metabolism. I'm not just talking about wild athletic fucking. High states of arousal and the physical changes that they produce—like faster breathing and higher blood pressure—can be very draining. Being fatigued or depleted can contribute to higher-than-average climax sensitivity.

In fact, the kind of food you eat can be more draining than energizing. Experts advise that a healthy diet, one that nourishes the body, can contribute to sexual well-being. Moderate exercise helps by stimulating the metabolic pathways you draw on during sex. That's why being overweight works against your sexual health. Consequently, if your health is less than stellar, you may be more likely to ejaculate involuntarily.

If you're trying to fix one cylinder of a V8 engine, it may never run smoothly at top speed if the other cylinders are weak.

Psychological Blocks

I'm taking the optimistic view, which works more than 95% of the time, that using the *Male Multiple Orgasm*'s techniques is simply a retraining process.

But I do want to alert you to the chance that something deeper in your mind can block your progress. There are some men who ejaculate too quickly at times because of unresolved psychological issues. Frequently, I encounter clients who used to have decent sexual stamina, but recently developed a problem due to work or relationship stress.

Many types of therapies can help address psychological problems. Possible therapies include personal therapy, Traumatic Incident Reduction, relationship counseling, and Tantric Sexual Healing.

If you're not making progress through the practices outlined in this book, or if you're having trouble staying the course with the program, consider consulting with a sex therapist or another appropriate professional.

CHAPTER 3

✧ *The Male Multiple Orgasm Formula*

Chapter 3 is all about what you'll gain from mastering Male Multiple Orgasm. First, I want to explain how the process works, why it's so important, and then go over the formula in detail.

MASTERING YOUR SEXUAL ENERGY

Male Multiple Orgasm is about mastering your own energy. I'm not referring to some obscure, New Age, airy-fairy imaginary phenomenon here. I'm talking about physical stuff you feel all the time. How do you become aware of being turned on, angry, nervous, or in love? Your internal energy causes sensations in your body. It's what acupuncturists and massage therapists work with every day.

It's All About Energy in Your Body

To be sure, at first, the energy that you'll be working with will seem far finer or subtler than a punch in the face or a mouth sucking you off. But, ultimately, subtle energy can be much more powerful than hard, fast pumping. That reminds me of a reserved female business associate at her first Tantra workshop. She experienced an hour of powerful, nonstop orgasmic vibrations shaking her whole body—just from a simple yoga breathing exercise.

Some say that women are generally more sensitive to energy. Maybe so, but of course guys feel it, too, some of us strongly. What causes goosebumps? A chill down your spine? Shivers or ticklishness? Or, more directly on our subject, how about that tingly warm feeling in your crotch when you see a very shapely female form swaying a wide path down the sidewalk?

When we refer to sexual energy, we mean the nervous stimulation and physical excitation that causes these feelings. You feel energy strongest just before an orgasm, thus the term "orgasmic energy." But it's all the same electrical or magnetic stuff in your body.

Regardless of what's causing your dissatisfaction with your lovemaking skills, energy is at the root of it. Male Multiple Orgasm techniques can help you conjure up orgasmic energy, heighten your senses of its effects, magnify its impact, and circulate it around the body.

Why bother learning how to channel energy? If all your sexual energy stays in vajra, the easiest direction for it to move is outward. And then you ejaculate. Spread that sexual energy around, and you feel great all over without a sudden big gush. As a result, you can have lots of little energy gushes, which get bigger and bigger and bigger, culminating in a long series of dry internal energy orgasms.

When the energy builds over and over inside, the sensations throughout your body can be much stronger than anything you've ever imagined.

Basic Sexual Energy Principles

You have so much exuberance bubbling inside you. Celebrate that wonderful orgasmic energy that makes you climax. If you can master the movement of this powerful energy, why limit these wonderful desires that spring to life? All you need to learn is how to direct that powerful urge to orgasm inward instead of outward to distribute and extend that energy that's ultimately so ecstatic.

Let me introduce you to some of the sexual energy mastery principles you'll find appearing in this book over and over. You'll learn to:

- Relax and go with the flow, allowing natural forces to run their course.
- Stop being inhibited or resisting healthy impulses.
- Be supremely conscious of everything while watching and enjoying.
- Be present in the moment and open your physical senses.
- Make love on multiple levels: sex, heart, and spirit.
- Focus on pleasure in the moment, not just on achieving the Big O.
- Know that you're responsible for your own pleasure and responses.
- Know what you desire, what your boundaries are, and voice them.
- Empty your mind of goals and anxieties, letting sex become a timeless, blissful meditation.
- Allow orgasm to become a sacred energy event SEPARATE from physical ejaculation.

Now doesn't that sound much better than learning tight control, always watching yourself, trying not to slip, and feeling bad when you do?

Your Energy Centers or Chakras

Many ancient cultures, particularly in the East, studied our subtle energies and devised methods to gain greater mastery over them. Common to many practices are the *chakras*, the Indian word for wheel. These are swirling energy centers or vortices inside your body, residing from the bottom of your spine to the top of your head. Though energy is energy, when it's generated in a specific chakra or settles in one, it feels unique and affects you differently than if it came from another place.

Why should you care? For two main reasons:

1) Most love partners want more than just a lust connection from the sex chakra. Merging energy at multiple chakras satisfies them immensely.

2) We'll use the *inner flute*, the invisible channel that connects the chakras, to move orgasmic energy away from your jewels so it won't make you ejaculate too soon.

Here are the common definitions of the seven chakras:

Chakra	Location	Function
1st	Perineum (base of spine)	Sex, survival
2nd	Belly (2 inches below navel)	Body, sensations
3rd	Solar Plexus	Power, will
4th	Heart	Love, compassion
5th	Throat	Creativity, expression
6th	Forehead (third eye)	Perception, consciousness
7th	Crown (top of head)	Divine connection

Energy Mastery Tools

Again and again, you'll receive advice in this book about using the "Four Cornerstones" of energy practice. The Four Cornerstones, which will become your key energy mastery tools, are:

- Presence (relaxation, mental focus, and concentration)
- Breath
- Sound
- Movement

These may seem like simple skills, and they are. When you use them consciously to get your sexual motor running, they can be ecstatic tools.

You might think that you already know what kind of physical attributes (breasts, rear, crotch, legs, long hair, etc.) turn you on. But those are external stimuli. The Four Cornerstones are internal tools you can use to energize your own pleasure and steer your own excitement.

In fact, we'll use these tools to simulate and ultimately create the feelings of orgasm: intense focus on sensations, deep breathing through the mouth, sinuous body vibrations with pelvic thrusts, and moans of pleasure. More importantly, we'll use the Four Cornerstones to spread the overwhelming excitation of sexual play away from the jewels.

Many of the exercises in the coming chapters directly utilize the Four Cornerstones.

WHY NOT EJACULATE?

I know I don't have to convince you that lasting longer is a great idea. But I do want to summarize in one place all the benefits of mastering Male Multiple Orgasm.

Voluntary Orgasm Means It's Up to You

Guys argue with me all the time about their confused idea that learning the energy mastery practice of Male Multiple Orgasm means not ejaculating. It doesn't have to be that way or any way. When you learn to go higher and higher forever, the simultaneous orgasm with your partner will be incredible. More importantly, when the ecstasy of the ride is greater than the brief release at the end, you may never want to let go so quickly again.

But the whole point of this program is that it will be up to you. Voluntary Orgasm Mastery is just that: you decide what you want, when you want it. And you have the skill to let it unfold according to your desires.

You can't experience the kind of ecstatic wave we're seeking here if you rush headlong toward orgasm or try to hold yourself back. You have to learn to relax into intense pleasure in order to go higher and higher.

Here's What You Lose by Ejaculating Too Quickly

Appreciate how powerfully this system of voluntary ejaculation may impact you. Here's what you could lose by ejaculating too quickly:

- Many women are multi-orgasmic because their energy isn't depleted by orgasm. You don't want to climax when she's ready for more.

- Most men's erections don't spring back to life quickly after ejaculation. As you age, it can even take a couple days to recover the ability to stay hard for long. Sex therapists call this the *refractory period*. So having an orgasm without ejaculating lets you repeat lovemaking as quickly and often as you want.

- Many men release lots of energy when they ejaculate, which makes them distant, sleepy, and exhausted. Don't ejaculate and you can stay energetic all night long.

- Many men lose the desire to continue making love after they ejaculate, suddenly ending the closeness and intimacy women crave. Some describe it as if a power switch was turned off.

- Many men shut down emotionally and mentally as well as physically, cutting off the communion at multiple levels that Male Multiple Orgasm can help you achieve.

Here's What You Gain by Not Ejaculating

Here is a list of all the benefits of learning Male Multiple Orgasm techniques. By choosing not to ejaculate, you can:

- Have hours of orgasmic pleasure instead of just a few seconds of intense release.

- Experience continuous peaks of ecstasy throughout your whole body.

- Stay connected with your partner longer, deeper, and at more levels.

- Promote health, vigor, and mental clarity by retaining your energy.

- Keep your entire body energized. (The Taoists believe that retaining your semen is highly nourishing and the key to longevity.)

- Fully satisfy your partner's previously unfulfilled sexual desires.
- Satisfy multiple partners one after the other without a break.
- Have bigger, stronger, longer-lasting orgasms when you finally choose to climax.

Wow! Just going over the list reminds me of the three main principles of Male Multiple Orgasm success: practice, practice, practice.

THE RAMPER FORMULA

The approach to learning Male Multiple Orgasm is called RAM-PER, which stands for:
- **R**elax
- **A**wareness
- **M**easure
- **P**ace yourself
- **E**nergy circulation
- **R**ide the wave.

Let me introduce you to the important aspects of each of these, so you'll know what you'll be practicing beginning in the next chapter.

R = Relax

You remember what normally happens to our bodies when we ejaculate? We tense and contract our pelvic muscles, especially around the rear, anus, stomach, and legs.

What do you think would happen if your muscles stayed completely flaccid (loose and relaxed) when you were highly excited? What would happen if you had no tension anywhere? You probably wouldn't ejaculate. This is the simplest technique and the hardest to learn.

If you can do this right now, then, congratulations, you've graduated from this program. But chances are it's going to take you awhile to master the simplicity of relaxing, just like it did for me.

But you are getting the point, right? A fundamental feature of the Male Multiple Orgasm is relaxation. Why? Because feeling calm and relaxed is the ideal state for S.E.X., or Subtle Energy eXchange. Tension blocks your blood flow and your feelings, not to mention the flow of orgasmic energy. When your channels are blocked, your energy collects in your jewels. As it builds up with nowhere else to go, you feel more and more pressure to ejaculate. The energy seeks the path of least resistance, out the tip of vajra. When you relax instead, open your inner channels, and let the energy move up your inner flute, you can more easily replace the rush to climax with the desire to savor the sensations in every moment.

S.E.X. is often much slower than the continuous, fast pumping you see in porno flicks. Just by going slower, you'll be more relaxed. How do you learn to relax while excited? First, by doing whatever you can to eliminate tension during sexual encounters. So much tension comes from performance anxiety or self-doubt. If you can get out of your head, you can relax much more easily. Often, this requires the kind of communication with your lover that we'll talk about later.

Being in your head means having expectations about what's going to happen and how you want to perform. THINKING sex is always less fulfilling than FEELING sex. Getting out of your head means letting go of so many of the worries that normally accompany sex, even with long-time partners. It means focusing on NOW instead of the slide show of pictures flashing inside your brain.

And it means dropping goals. If you plan to make your sweetie orgasm big time, or last two hours instead of your record of one hour, or be twice as turned on as last time, then you're setting up mental goals. Maybe this works well for you in business. But when it comes to managing energy inside, it can work against you by taking your awareness out of the moment.

Remember that energy flows where attention goes. If you have any of these goals in your mind, you'll be comparing your performance against that picture you created in your head. This is the exact anatomy of tension. The Male Multiple Orgasm, contradictory as it sounds, is based on letting go of the need to control the outcome of your lovemaking. Your aim instead is to relax and enjoy. Once you learn how to stay loose, deeply comfortable, and drift with the natural flow of energy, you'll soar with pleasure instead of losing it.

How can you learn to relax? In the 'Solo Exercises' chapter that follows, I'll show you physical techniques that assist your mental relaxation. You'll learn how to squeeze your muscles to relax them, especially your sexual muscles. I'll remind you to keep your tongue on the roof of your mouth so you don't tense up one of the most important parts of your body, your jaw.

Foremost amongst these relaxation techniques is breathing. Remember what happens to your breath when you climax? You start breathing rapidly and panting. What do you think would happen if you knew how to breathe deeply and slowly even while being swamped with ecstatic feelings? You got it: you would be washed inside and out with orgasmic energy without releasing your precious little swimmers.

Westerners breathe shallowly and unconsciously. Contrast that with Yoga masters. Some are so aware that they can shut their breathing down to almost nothing and stay in a state of suspended animation for extended periods. Don't get me wrong, I'm not trying to convert you into any spiritual practice other than sex as a delightfully refreshing focused sensual meditation. But do you get that the Male Multiple Orgasm is more like floating with the current than fighting your way upstream?

Relax, and your sexual energy will set you free. You can quote me on that.

A = Awareness

If you're thinking about making your partner climax while holding back your own ejaculation, your awareness will be consumed with thoughts of orgasm. Male Multiple Orgasm helps you generate incredible mutual orgasms, but without directly targeting them. As mentioned earlier, your focus needs to be on pleasure in the moment. If you can appreciate how great vajra feels now, you'll be more willing and able to relax and go slow.

To become pleasure-centered, you need to heighten your *sensate focus*. Sensate focus means tuning in to all your senses: taste, touch, sight, sound, and smell. It means delighting in every sight, basking in every fragrance, and savoring every sensation. If you become more sensitive to everything that's happening all around and all over your body, you won't have the common situation of untrained lovers: total focus on the jewels. Instead, you can distribute that delicious energy to all your chakras.

As we just discussed, relaxation helps you awaken your senses and embrace the sensations in every moment. If you haven't learned to go with the flow and be in the moment without goals or expectations, mental tension will shift your attention away from the feelings of the moment. The relaxation and awareness exercises in the next chapter may not start very sexually, but I hope you'll soon see how essential they are to your success.

More importantly, though, most guys who don't last very long aren't good at recognizing the internal signals that could warn of impending ejaculation. If you learn to register every little nuance of every little feeling, going slowly and digesting all the energy, then you're less likely to trip over the point of no return. When you're enjoying every breath, sound, and movement, you'll be supremely conscious of your own level of excitement. And you'll be able to respond to that excitement before it becomes too hard to manage, pushing you over the cliff into a gushing plunge down the chasm.

How can you manage your energy flows if you're not completely tuned in to them? You can't. Make it your mission to focus on your feelings. Being present in the moment is one of the vital Four Cornerstones of energy mastery and directly impacts your ability to relax. So, heighten your senses, feel your feelings, enjoy your pleasure with no agenda, and you'll gradually learn to stay out of your head and into your body.

By the way, due to tension and social pressure, many of us find ourselves partying with recreational drugs and alcohol. Again, I don't intend to moralize, so let's just be pragmatic. Although some believe that drugs and alcohol can slow ejaculatory response, they'll also keep you from developing the body awareness that will allow you to change your lovemaking stamina permanently. Getting high may feel good temporarily, but it makes it much harder to master the timing of your orgasms. Thinking about other things—like football or your latest weekend project—can be counterproductive, too, for the same reason.

More awareness is the prescription for more manageable pleasure, not less.

M = Measure Your Level of Arousal

By now, you've heard again and again that you have to tune in to your senses and sensations. So what do you do with this sharpened awareness?

The M in RAMPER means to monitor and measure your level of arousal. Arousal awareness is complex, with lots of subtlety. It's more like a rainbow than black and white. The forces that turn us on aren't always obvious in the moment, and change from time to time. So the M step is all about learning to read yourself, so you can know where you're at right now.

This is not just a scientific experiment. Rather, it's a technique to help you become more sensitive to what makes you excited. If you know where your excitement level is and what causes it, then you can play spontaneously while stretching out your enjoyment and that of your partner. And you can take responsibility for your own pleasure, guiding your lovemaking so that you get really turned on and stay there, without going too far too fast.

Many sex therapists recommend using a 10-point scale for monitoring your level of arousal during practice and sex play. This is one of the main things we'll be focusing on in the coming exercises. (By the way, level of arousal may not correspond to the strength of your erection at any given moment.)

Here's my version of the 10-point arousal scale:

0 = Rest state with no arousal

1 = Twinge at base of penis

2 = Occasional little tingles of pleasure

3 = Starting to warm up and feel good

4 = Steady low-level arousal

5 = Pleasure surges feel really good

6 = Metabolism increases, feeling focused and not wanting to stop

7 = Continuous rush of pleasure, fast breathing

8 = Buzzing inside, electrical current running

9 = Intense pleasure, involuntary contractions

9.9 = Point of no return, emission phase begins

10 = Ejaculation at expulsion phase

As you practice, you'll learn to measure your level of arousal as it climbs toward 9.9, the point of no return. You know the feeling of time stopping, like the movie clip that suddenly goes into slow motion as you watch the car careen over the cliff? You've been enjoying yourself immensely, maybe even feeling far from ejaculating, when all of a sudden you feel those involuntary contractions around your prostate and you know you're gonna let go. That's the often uninvited guest, 9.9, buddy.

A major part of self-monitoring during your individual practices will be learning how close you can go to 9.9 without going over the edge. This is a tough thing to accept, guys, but you're going to have to play with yourself over and over again as you learn this system. Bummer!

By the way, I don't refer to such divine play as masturbation, which has hidden and dirty connotations. I prefer to call it *self-pleasuring*, which is a wonderful and sacred thing. If you don't already, you're going to have to learn to enjoy giving yourself pleasure. Get used to the idea.

P = Pace Yourself

OK, you've relaxed. You've become more sensitive. You've measured how good it feels. Will these things change your stamina dramatically? Well, maybe. But really the RAM part of RAMPER is simply vital preparation for the P step. P stands for Pacing yourself.

No, I take that back. P stands for Pleasure. If your focus is on pleasure, not orgasm, then you won't be rushing headlong toward a destination. You won't be in a race toward the finish line. You won't have a schedule to meet. You'll just slow down and enjoy. That's a big part of pacing. And if you learn how to make the pleasure you enjoy greater than any quick dribble you've ever experienced, you'll want to pace yourself for more, More, and MORE!

Later we'll get into talking about what to do with partners who get so excited that they don't let you pace yourself. Sure, that happens and in their rush to orgasm they'll drag you over the precipice. And if you both climax together, wonderful! But when push comes to shove, what most lovers really want is for you to go all night. Eventually, with the right kind of guidance, they'll listen to reason. I'll show you later how to solicit their ecstatic participation.

Again, Male Multiple Orgasm is all about learning to ride the edge, that fine line between absorbing all the pleasure you can take, and taking too much all at once and ejaculating. Like I mentioned before, you'll rarely hear me talk about control for this reason. Control makes you tight, tense, and rigid, the opposite of relaxation. Control requires you to set standards and watch yourself all the time, stopping the flow of your energy to pull yourself back from the brink. Riding the edge is relaxed, more like skipping from wave top to wave top than fighting the surf with strong steering motions and lots of big throttle adjustments. When you ride the wave, you relax, savor the sweet sensations, and gradually and gently add little bits of arousal as you can take it.

The key to "P = Pace Yourself" is also about two more P words: peaking and plateauing. Peaking means adjusting the stimuli that give you sudden surges of arousal so you come back down without going over the top. If you graphed peaking like Figure 3, it would look like a steep ascent and then a steep descent. Which is where it got its name.

Plateauing is the advanced skill that you learn once you get good at peaking. As Figure 4 shows, plateauing is where you learn how to maintain a high level of arousal for a while without backing off.

Now you see what relaxing, awareness, and measuring will do for you? They're the essential tools you use to recognize when you're reaching a peak that's too close to the point of no return. This heightened sensitivity in that moment lets you slow down or stop soon enough. When you master getting close to 9.9 and backing off,

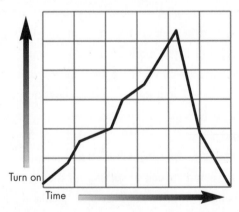

Figure 3: Peaking

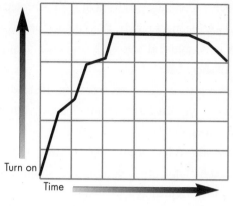

Figure 4: Plateauing

then you'll learn even subtler adjustments so can enjoy plateaus for long periods of time. Some call these *valley orgasms* because their arousal curve flattens out instead of peaking up sharply.

Oh yeah, there's an important section in Chapter 5 called "Interrupting Ejaculation" which assists you with learning to peak. It will show you more than a half-dozen physical techniques to stop losing it when you stray too close to 9.9. Frankly, these aren't my favorite techniques for two reasons. First, stopping something from happening isn't really one of the more useful energy tools. Second, I have to admit that I'm not too good at them. Maybe they'll help you, so I've included the whole story. But for me, Male Multiple Orgasm is more about energy circulation than interrupting the emission phase.

E = Energy Circulation

E stands for Energy, for circulating it away from your jewels. But it could also stand for the Ecstasy that results from filling up with this great stuff that can give you dry full-body orgasms. In fact, the E is central to Male Multiple Orgasm since it's really about S.E.X.—which is Subtle Energy eXstacy.

Because most of us are programmed to rush toward the Big O, we come into the arena of love play tempted to release our sexual energy through explosive jewel orgasms. It's what books, flicks, and locker room talk glorify. That's the accepted concept of good sex in most people's minds. Who among us has been fortunate enough to be initiated reverently and openly into the higher dimensions of sacred sex?

So here's a vital part of your initiation: Instead of shooting for the Big O as your arousal builds, spread your energy up, around, and throughout your body away from your jewels, allowing it to carry you to higher and higher levels of pleasure. Not only will it feel ecstatic, you'll be able to last and last and last, since you won't be depleting your energy.

How do you do it? Simply explained, you channel your sexual energy up your inner flute from your first chakra (the sex center at the base of the spine) so vajra doesn't explode in a gush of ejaculation. You redirect your orgasmic energy primarily by using the Four Cornerstones: presence, breath, sound, and movement. Admittedly, learning it may not be as simple as describing it. For sure, it took me months. That's a big reason why there are so many exercises is this book.

For some, it may come naturally. My friend, Rick, for example, knew how to run energy instinctively as a teenager. Of course, everyone (his big brother paramount among them) told him he was weird. So instead of acting "crazy," he suppressed his natural ability for years. Fortunately, today he's using his natural talent and is one of the best and longest-lasting lovers I've ever met. (He asked me to put his phone number here with the message "For a good time call Rick..." but I didn't think you guys would particularly like that.)

Once you learn to circulate (move, run, channel) energy, you experience amazingly powerful sensations. Imagine what it feels like when that excitation making vajra pulse and throb infuses other parts of your body. So, the E of RAMPER is to channel your orgasmic energy elsewhere in your body. What do you do with it? Well, first off, move it to your heart and energize your love center.

You know how women are always squawking about finding a sensitive guy? They'll love you when your heart is activated by sexual energy. And when one of your chakras is really turned on, you can flood your partner's equivalent chakra with your energy. Circulating energy then becomes a sharing exercise as well as an internal one. Some say it will fuel your brain with cosmic energy and give you both psychedelic visions.

My friend Doc Steven is the master of this. I asked him once, after observing his love exploits for over a year, when was the last time he came. He had to think about it a while and said it was about three years previously. "How do you do it?" I asked. His answer: "I love women so much, that it's totally natural for me to move those sexual juices to my heart, and then I love them more. And they go wild for a compassionate, caring, sensitive lover who only wants them to feel ecstasy above all else."

So he turns his heart on with some of his sexual energy, not just his vajra.

We've talked about the Four Cornerstones, the orgasmic keys of presence, breath, sound, and movement, to amplify your energy and feel more passion. These are the primary tools of running energy: visualizing that juice spreading inside, breathing deep in the belly, moaning with pleasure, rocking your hips, and squeezing your sexual muscles (which pumps energy up your inner flute). After lots of practice, I've really proven to myself that uttering love sounds releases energy that would otherwise just settle in my jewels. If you're the macho silent type, it may take some getting used to. But it's well worth it. Believe me, your partners will love to hear how turned on you are, too.

As discussed previously, the net impact of running energy is learning to separate ejaculation from orgasm. When you're relaxed inside and super turned on, the contractions around your prostate that initiate the emission of semen don't have to be activated. When the energy becomes intense, you can still have those powerful pelvic muscle contractions that feel so wonderful.

That's what causes a dry orgasm: a long series of slow pleasurable spasms without ejaculating and with a rush of energy. I call these *implosive orgasms* because the energy gets pumped back inside so it can circulate over and over again.

Now here's the best news of all: When you have a dry implosive orgasm, all of a sudden your arousal decreases dramatically. On the other side of that peak, you're suddenly less sensitive, so you can stroke faster and let the excitement build again. By circulating sexual energy around your body while peaking, being on the verge of 9.9 comes and goes. Done right, it can make your love stamina virtually unlimited.

R = Ride the Orgasmic Wave

When you retain your energy inside, your pleasure rises to higher and higher levels. That's why the acronym RAMPER is so apt, describing how your pleasure ramps up. Those who ejaculate quickly never experience these escalating plateaus. You never develop your capacity to absorb more and more pleasure. When you finally do, it feels like ecstatic waves surging inside. What was a 9 on the arousal scale a half-hour ago now becomes just a 6. And when you get back up to 9, it's so much more. That's what the final R is about, Riding the orgasmic wave.

Here's what my beautiful wife, Jeffre, says about sex...

> "Straight pumping is boring and makes me numb. I
> really love to go slow, like pump, pump, pump, and relax. I
> just let the energy wash over me. Then a few more strokes
> and the orgasmic waves, little implosive orgasms, roll
> through me. By doing this over and over again and again,
> I eventually get to higher and higher plateaus."

You see how Male Multiple Orgasm is ecstatic when all the pieces come together? You relax and heighten your awareness of your senses to open yourself to subtle energy. By measuring your arousal, you learn to pace, peak, and plateau. This builds up intense energy, which you circulate around your body instead of exploding with a quick release. Then the wave takes you, and you just float.

When your energy rises to your spiritual centers, the higher chakras, you'll find a natural calming and blissful feeling engulfing you. It's as if your orgasmic energy is fueling your soul's psychic nature. This is why we call S.E.X. sexual meditation. Some describe this as feeling like a hollow bamboo with a never-ending supply of energy running between the earth and sky through the body.

S.E.X. uses the same body parts and erogenous zones you see in X-rated flicks. But the actions inside and out are vastly different. S.E.X., being as much spiritual as it is physical, looks slow and conscious. It's not focused on orgasm, but on building pleasure and making it last forever. This takes harmony, openness, and lots of communication between partners.

As you play more and more with the same partner, you'll undoubtedly learn moves that please and cues that tip you when to use them. When you meditate sexually together, you must each be totally centered and responsible for your own personal experience. Lovers want different things at different times. Even the most skilled lovers can't always predict the whims and changes erupting in spontaneous love play. So both partners must be tuned in to themselves as well as to each other. This only works when you welcome guidance from your lover, whether verbal or subtle, and truly become a team that's totally in sync with each other.

If you're single and trying to attract a partner, or have one who's into a totally different experience, riding the kind of orgasmic wave I've just described may conjure up problems. There are different styles of lovers and they are not all compatible with each other. Later, I'll show you how to motivate, guide, and coach potential or current sex partners so you can build the kind of love team I'm encouraging. But this may not be what some lovers want and you may have to simply accept that they're not for you.

CHAPTER 4

✧ *Solo Prep*

Chapter 4 is the first of two chapters that present solo exercises. These are the exercises you do on your own, even if you have a love partner. This chapter concentrates on you: preparing yourself, developing basic sensual skills, and building the foundation you'll need to become an Orgasm Master.

PRACTICE GUIDELINES

First, I want to give you some general guidelines for practicing. If you have a partner, now is a good time to let them know what's going on. Next, I want to make a few comments about the least effective methods for success, namely, desensitizing vajra's quick response. Then I'll show you how to practice RAM, the first three parts of RAMPER. We'll start by relaxing, move to ways to heighten your senses (awareness), and focus in a big way on learning to measure your arousal.

So that you can begin daily practice, I've included some vital exercises to strengthen your pelvic (PC) muscles. Start doing these exercises right away because the strength of your PC muscles will become a vital part of your orgasm mastery.

An Exercise Program

First of all, Male Multiple Orgasm (MMO) is an exercise program for much more than your PC muscles. It's like going to the gym to work various muscle groups. Of course, in this case you'll be developing your sexual reflexes, which are defined by RAMPER. Plan for the long gradual approach as opposed to the one-shot deal.

Above all, take your time. It doesn't matter how fast you work through these exercises, as long as you keep at it for 30 to 60 minutes every day or two, or as close to that as you can manage. To change your sexual life dramatically, you'll need to stay with this program for several months. No one can guarantee that you'll change a lifelong pattern overnight.

If you went to the gym to start building your upper body, would you start with the maximum weight that Mr. Universe can lift? Of course not. Even he started slowly and gradually. If you push yourself to the limit, you could strain yourself at the beginning. That kind of short-term setback won't prevent you from succeeding all by itself, but you could get so demoralized that you'd quit. So start slow and easy.

Since we're on the subject, remember that we modern Westerners are preconditioned to expect instant gratification. You know what I mean: "I want it and I want it now." I can't blame us for having this mentality, living as we do bombarded with modern media, technology, and advertising. It just doesn't work very well in the bedroom. Maybe that's part of the reason why those of us sensitive souls who haven't given and received sufficient sexual pleasure tend to climax quickly. We want all the pleasure immediately!

Slow Down

Your first global assignment is to slow down. Please don't start out expecting instant results. You might have some amazing changes quickly. Many do, but don't bank on it. Expectations will just add to your anxiety level and decrease the first step of RAMPER, namely to relax. Instead, start slowly, feel good about doing a little and then a little bit more, and good things will happen eventually.

For the most part, these exercises build on each other. There's no gospel about the perfect order, but I've arranged them in a sequence that makes sense about what to master first. The learning strategy here is a gradient, developing basic skills first, then building more and more complex actions on top of them with small steps. For example, you need to relax before practicing peaking because if you don't relax at just the right moment, you'll blow right past the point of no return.

Even after you become an Orgasm Master, you'll want to continue doing some MMO practices regularly to stay in shape. From other exercises, you'll get a kind of breakthrough, which you can then incorporate into your life as a natural part of your sensuous play. So, your exercise program will go through phases which I'll explain as we progress.

Take an Easy-Going Approach

Do you understand that you need to begin this program with an easy-going approach? That means relaxing into the moment and just accepting what happens at each step along the way.

Don't force yourself or try to rush your progress, and don't beat yourself up if things don't go according to some schedule you make up in your head. It may sound like a complete paradox, but believe me, to go as fast as possible, drop all those goals about how fast you want to get where you're going. Just take it step-by-step.

And know you need to allow room for error. If you create a plan and define stringent performance standards, you'll put pressure on yourself to perform. We've already covered how much that can contribute to involuntary ejaculation. So drop those mental pictures, too, OK?

To create the right kind of practice setting, you'll want a stress-free environment with privacy and without fear of being interrupted. Find or create a clean, comfortable room where you feel relaxed. A room with a music system or where you can lug a boom box will help. Energy practices benefit from having the right kind of mood music.

For example, use meditative music for the relaxing and awareness exercises at RAM (Relax, Awareness, Measure), and more rhythmic sounds for the sensual exercises at PER (Pace, Energy, Ride the wave). The Resources section at the back of this book and at my website www.TantraAtTahoe.com/resources.htm have some examples of my favorite music.

You may need to block out some time every day or two in your weekly schedule so you remember to practice often and maintain your focus. If you can't make this appointment with yourself every time you've scheduled, don't sweat it. Just make sure you practice several times a week. A half-hour a week just isn't enough. And by the way, except for the sexual muscle exercises, try not to squeeze in your practice between pressing deadlines while you're on the run. The less time crunch and mental pressure, the better you'll be able to focus.

Basically, just have fun and enjoy yourself. Don't turn a program to build sexual ecstasy into arduous work. Heck, in a few pages I'm going to ask you to pleasure vajra. You want that to become a chore? I hope not.

To Climax or Not to Climax

Yes, your goal is for you to master orgasms and separate them from ejaculating. But this whole pursuit is about pleasure and enjoyment. The ends definitely do not justify harsh, unpleasant means. So, after a solo practice session of stimulating yourself, you may want to climax. I'm not going to preach about this in the instructions for every exercise. Take the following guidelines to heart right now.

You may have so much juice and sexual energy built up that an explosive release may be just what your body needs. Wonderful! Releasing the tension may help you last longer next time. Good! You may be so turned on that you feel you've got to let go now. Fine! Or you may enjoy it so much that you feel you deserve a reward. Great, go for it! Just remember to appreciate your fantastic, God-given talent for giving yourself pleasure. It's a gift.

Taoist texts emphasize how much energy you lose by releasing your seed. They preach that ejaculating too often is bad for you. One of their ancient texts, *The Secrets Of The Jade Bedroom*, (as quoted on page 222 of *Sexual Secrets* by Nik Douglas and Penny Slinger, Destiny Books, Rochester VT 2000), recommends a healthy ejaculation frequency of wet orgasm for men of various ages. If you're a healthy 15-year-old, it suggests you can ejaculate twice a day. As you age, here are the book's general guidelines for a healthy male:

When you're...	You can ejaculate once every...
30	1 day
40	3 days
50	5 days
60	10 days
70	30 days

If you're sick, highly emotional, or under undue stress, the book recommends releasing only half as often as indicated. Regardless of what you choose to do at any time, let's face a bottom-line reality right now. You WILL go over the top accidentally and ejaculate more times than you intend. As you learn to dance and flow with this powerful force, you'll slip past the point of no return. If you don't, you're not getting close enough. So expect some unintentional wet spots before you master prolonging your ecstasy.

When you do ejaculate unexpectedly, don't beat yourself up. Enjoy it. That's what this whole game of sex is about, right?

Partner Briefing

If you have one primary long-term partner or several lovers that you're intimate with, I strongly recommend you brief them on what you're doing here. This is partly because secrecy can create tension that contributes to involuntary explosions of the seminal variety. This chapter and the next discuss solo pleasuring because refining your arousal pattern is exciting enough in private. If someone else is present, it could be too exciting at first, or too embarrassing to relax.

Before you've begun your practice program, I don't suggest you try to cover everything in your partner "briefing." If you've already explained that you're embarking on this program, that's great. You've started as a partnership and have already talked about it. If not, asking your lover to check our free Online Guided Tour about premature ejaculation at TantraAtTahoe.com would be a good foundation.

Regardless, you want to alert your partner or partners that you're starting a series of private exercises, so they'll understand what you're up to when you disappear every day or so.

If your partner isn't yet aware of what you're doing, here are some suggestions about how to approach your talk:

- "I found an interesting website recently about improving our lovemaking. It's based on Tantra, an ancient spiritual practice that uses sexual energy to raise consciousness."
- "I recently bought an interesting book about improving our lovemaking and extending my sexual stamina, based on ancient sexual energy exercises."
- "I want you to know that I'll be doing some solo sensuous exercises in private for a few weeks. They're designed to help my personal development. I'll let you know how it's progressing and hope to get you involved soon."

The more forthright you're comfortable being, the better. If you want to be more specific at this stage, you can also say:

- "The book I'm reading is called *Male Multiple Orgasm*. I really believe that I'll be able to lengthen our lovemaking by using this program. Are you interested in reading about what I'll be practicing?"

If this is difficult for you, now might be a good time to talk to a sex therapist or counselor about changing your relationship dynamics. The more support you get from your partner, the faster your results will be.

DESENSITIZING

Desensitizing means using products or techniques that make vajra less responsive temporarily. You probably get spam emails about all sorts of bogus offers—pills to make you last forever or creams to add 6 inches to your penis. Experts report these methods usually don't help premature ejaculation much in the long-term. In fact, the whole idea is repugnant to an evolved lover who aims to heighten his senses, not reduce them. But it's understandable that you'd want to know if, when, and how desensitizing works. In fact, it may even help a given situation in the short-term. So here is advice about some methods that are available:

Pre-Masturbation

Pre-masturbation means having sex alone about two to four hours before the big event. The method is based on the fact that most of us are less sensitive and have less desire after ejaculating.

The problem with this technique is that your level of arousal is only part of what contributes to involuntary ejaculation. If you're still mentally absorbed with lasting longer, you'll likely only gain a few minutes. It's true, it may take you a bit longer the second time before you approach arousal level 9.9. But if you're not intimately aware of your level of arousal at each moment, you may have the same trouble slipping over the edge once you arrive. If you haven't mastered peaking just short of the point of no return, you're still likely to lose it quickly.

If pre-masturbation doubles your time of lasting from five minutes to ten minutes, you might consider it progress. I don't have a problem with that while you're learning the Male Multiple

Orgasm techniques. But face it, it's far short of what true Orgasm Mastery will allow you to do.

Creams

Desensitizing creams are products that claim to lessen the sensations felt by men during sexual union (intercourse) so that they can last longer. I haven't tried them, but it makes sense from a purely physical point of view, doesn't it? A shot of Novocain in vajra would be enough to scare anyone away from slipping when you don't want to. But if one of these creams works on you and makes sex less pleasurable by decreasing stimulation, it's kind of a self-defeating, win-lose victory. It might feel good in your mind if you can last longer, but if it's only fun for your partner, how often will you want to do it? Wouldn't you rather have more intense sensations lasting for hours? Sounds like a much better win-win to me.

Pills

Some medications reduce vajra's sensitivity. Some doctors prescribe tranquilizer-type drugs to reduce a guy's sensitivity. From surfing the net in places like the Yahoo group about premature ejaculation, I've read that these medications aren't too reliable. Plus, they're expensive and probably have side effects. I'd much rather have a free, natural solution that's under my command. Wouldn't you?

Condoms

If you're careful about safe sex these days, you're aware that condoms, used properly, help protect against STDs (sexually transmitted diseases) and unwanted pregnancies. Obviously, a layer of latex covering vajra's sensitive skin reduces the amount of stimulation you receive during sex. Some men find that wearing a condom helps them last longer by lowering their arousal. I've even heard that some men use two or three to decrease their sensitivity even more.

Again, it can take you longer to get to the point of no return this way, which is good. But when you arrive at the edge of the cliff with those wonderful feelings swirling around you, will you be able to handle it any better? I find not. So you'll still need Male Multiple Orgasm techniques.

RELAXATION

Calm and relaxed is the ideal state for long-lasting lovemaking. That way, there'll be no tension to prevent the natural flow of orgasmic energy. When you relax and awaken your senses, which we'll work on next, you can more easily replace the rush to climax with the desire to savor each sensation every moment.

Mastery Begins with R

Your ejaculation mastery exercises begin with the R of RAMPER, for relaxing. Why is this vital? Remember, letting go too soon is often triggered by tension in the pelvis, butt, or mind.

Several exercises follow that can help you teach your body to relax on command. Though each one is different, they're all basically simple. Try them and see what works for you.

Exercise: Corpse Posture

There's a yoga position called the corpse posture, which is a good place to start when making relaxation a sensual discipline. Here's how you do it:

1) Lie down on your back and close your eyes. Use a pillow under your knees and neck if needed for comfort.

2) Spread your legs slightly and let your arms fall away from your body with your palms up.

3) Imagine the weight of your body pressing down into the earth while being entirely supported all around.

4) Just let go of all the tension in your body, allowing all your muscles to completely relax. Let your mind float free.

5) Focus on the slow, steady natural rhythm of your breathing. Let that be the only thing you're aware of while your mind relaxes.

6) Just float this way for 20 minutes while you witness what your mind and body experience.

You can practice this regularly before other exercises or anytime you want to dissolve any of the stresses that you accumulate during normal life. Some people find that recording these instructions on an audio tape and listening to them in their own voice helps them relax more and faster.

Exercise: Muscle Relaxation

In this exercise, you'll systematically isolate, tense, and then relax each muscle group in your body, starting with your toes. When muscles are tense, it's common for most of us to clench our jaw muscles. So a good tip for all the exercises in this book, especially the relaxation ones, is to keep your tongue on your palate lightly touching the roof of your mouth. Then you can't unconsciously bite down hard or gnash your teeth.

To do Muscle Relaxation:

1) Lie down and close your eyes in the corpse posture or any other way you feel comfortable. (If the corpse posture isn't comfortable, find a lying or sitting position where you can totally relax.)

2) Focus your awareness on your toes, tense them tightly for a moment, and then relax them for several breaths.

3) Focus your awareness on your feet, tense them tightly for a moment, and then relax them for several breaths.

4) Continue doing the same with your lower legs, thighs, jewels, butt, stomach, lower back, chest, upper back, hands, forearms, upper arms, shoulders, neck, and jaw.

5) If you feel tension remaining anywhere, repeat the cycle until you feel relaxed all over.

6) Take a few moments just breathing gently and feel the complete sense of relaxation sink in deeply.

With enough relaxation practice, your body will remember the sensation and you'll be able to go into this floating state quickly and easily at will. In Chapter 6, we'll discuss other relaxation techniques, such as massage, which require a partner.

Exercise: Sitting Meditation

My intention is not to convert you into some kind of modern yogi or spiritual guru. But to be completely honest, meditation is one of the most powerful ways to relax. So I'm including this optional exercise, which I hope you'll try at least a few times to see how powerful it can be.

Meditation is simply sitting and emptying the mind. Since you can't force thoughts away, this is more challenging than it sounds. Gurus have developed many meditation techniques that can help you quiet the mind and enter a "no mind" condition. I've tried many and they all seek to create a deep inner peace filled with stillness.

The simple method I present here just guides you to watch your breath. It's good preparation for what's coming, because conscious breathing is one of the energy mastery skills used in the exercises that follow.

1) Sit in a comfortable position in a quiet, uninterrupted space. Turn off your phone, pager, and TV.

2) The classic posture is the lotus position, with one leg crossed over the other. I can't get all the way into it myself, and it may not be easy for you either. Get as close as you can and try to sit upright. I use a *zafu*, a round Japanese meditation pillow that's rather firm and shaped like a fat pancake. It makes sitting easier by keeping my pelvis higher than my semi-crossed legs. You can also meditate sitting straight in a comfortable chair or on a sofa.

3) Meditation is not doing anything—it's simply being. So don't set any goals or preconceptions of what's going to happen. Just sit for a moment and relax.

4) As you settle in to a comfortable state, you'll undoubtedly discover that your mind is busy. Don't do anything about it, but just let it happen. Witness ideas floating by like clouds in the wind.

5) To quiet the mind without force, watch your breath coming in and out. Don't change your breathing consciously, just pay attention to it.

6) You'll probably find your concentration wandering away from your breath. Don't beat yourself up, because it's natural. When you realize you've strayed, just come back to watching your breath.

7) Gurus advise 15 minutes sitting like this twice a day, morning and afternoon. Since you shouldn't be watching the clock, I guess you're supposed to set a timer. I usually just remain still until I relax and my mind settles.

If you incorporate regular meditation into your life, you'll find that it's a great way to relieve stress. It's supposed to be good for you physically and mentally, too. We're mostly concerned here with how it helps you with MMO techniques. All I can say is that tension makes you ejaculate more easily and relaxation is vital to lasting longer. Meditation practice isn't essential, but it can be a great tool to release tension and help you relax.

Exercise: Deep Belly Breathing

When the average person gets close to orgasm, their breath becomes shorter and faster, maybe even with uncontrollable panting. So, one of the best ways to relax when excited is to learn to breathe slower and deeper. Further, it helps to interrupt the stress response you may experience during exciting or anxious moments of lovemaking.

Most of us take breathing for granted. We breathe shallowly as a rule. We could all benefit from mastering the art of Deep Belly Breathing: relaxed, through the mouth, and deep into the stomach. This kind of full breathing lowers the heart rate and can help dissipate the tension of arousal. Breathing through the mouth is more physical and sensual as opposed to breathing through the nose, which tends to put the attention in the mind.

To practice Deep Belly Breathing:

1) Lie down in a comfortable position like the corpse posture and close your eyes.

2) Remain completely still, relaxing all your muscles, especially your anal and genital muscles. Press your tongue gently against the roof of your mouth to keep your jaw relaxed.

3) Without consciously changing anything, watch how rapidly you breathe and feel how deeply each breath goes.

4) To begin Deep Belly Breathing, open your mouth and breathe rhythmically, all the way down into your stomach. Imagine that your belly is an empty balloon that fills and empties with each relaxing breath.

5) Put your hand on your belly and feel it move in and out as you breathe. If your hand isn't moving, consciously force the air down deeper. Make sure that it's your breath moving your hand, not the extension of your stomach muscles.

6) To take it a step further, imagine your breath going down into your pelvis—washing, cleansing, and stimulating. As your breath trickles out, imagine it leaving every muscle totally relaxed.

Slow Deep Belly Breathing is an essential component of Male Multiple Orgasm. Later, you'll need this technique to channel sexual energy away from your jewels in order to make love longer. Practice this as long and as often as you need. Continue until you can easily and rhythmically fall into slow, relaxing belly breathing through your mouth.

BUILD YOUR SEXUAL MUSCLES

As with any physical calisthenics, improved tone gives you better muscle control. When a muscle is weak, it feels like mush after a little exercise, whether at the gym or in the sack. If you're not in charge of what your sexual muscles are doing when you're making love or getting oral sex, then you're missing a critical tool in your arsenal to avoid exploding unexpectedly. I like to call them sexual muscles because they're vital to pumping sexual energy away from your jewels. In other words, this is a big key to Orgasm Mastery.

Another Vital Part of Relaxing

There's another vital part of the R for relaxing in RAMPER that has to do with the sexual muscles in your pelvis around vajra and the twins. But it all starts with healthy, well-toned pelvic (PC) muscles that can completely relax when you want them to, or clamp tight for a couple minutes when you so desire. Start a daily routine of exercises to strengthen your PC muscles now so you'll have them at your disposal when you need them.

Strong Sexual Muscles Are Way Handy

The muscles in your pelvis pulse rhythmically during sexual union (intercourse), and rapidly during the expulsion phase of ejaculation. If you strengthen and tone them sufficiently, you can learn to regulate their contractions, consciously making them slower. This expands your orgasmic sensations during lovemaking and spreads your pleasure out. Most significantly, it reduces the urge to have a wet climax before you're ready.

But wait, there's even more good news. If you develop strong sexual muscles, you can have stronger erections, more powerful orgasms, and bounce your hard vajra on your lover's G-Spot. That's right, you can't give her G-Spot a good bounce without sexual muscles of steel.

Some believe that these exercises also massage your prostate and keep that vital organ healthier—a great side benefit. As far as I'm concerned, that's all well and good as long as it gives you greater control over the ejaculation response, which it does.

Later on, strong sexual muscles will come in handy, too. Using your internal PC muscles is a vital part of the E in RAMPER. Remember, E stands for energy, and your pelvic strength is an important method of spreading the sexual energy of explosive orgasms up throughout the body.

Because toning the muscles at the floor of your pelvis is critical to this program and doesn't happen overnight, I want you to decide to add some of these exercises to your daily routine now. Then, as you get stronger, you'll gradually learn how to relax them more and more, and you'll be able to use them to pump energy when you need to.

Call Me PC for Short

So what exactly are these magical sexual muscles hiding deep inside your crotch? I've been calling them PC, which is short for pubococcygeus.

I know that's a mouthful, but it's easy to identify. Put one of your hands on your pubic bone, the inside one that's above vajra at the bottom of your tummy. Now reach around behind and put your other hand near the top of your crack at the very bottom of your spine. That's your coccyx (tailbone). The PC muscle snakes down around your rosetta and jewels and connects these two bones plus your sitting bones and legs.

It's even more important to identify the muscle from the inside. It's the one you tighten when you want to squeeze out the last few drops of pee or need to stop midstream. Try squeezing it now. Did you make vajra jump? If you can't isolate it, take a break and go the bathroom right now. Start peeing and stop in the middle. When you're finished, try to squeeze out the last few drops. The muscle you used to stop midstream and squeeze at the end is your PC.

By the way, if you've been involved in a woman's recovery after childbirth, you've probably heard of *kegels*. These are similar exercises developed in 1952 by a gynecologist, Dr. Arnold Kegel. He taught women to flex their PC muscles to restore tone after the trauma of childbirth and help them regain control of their urinary reflexes.

We guys are more interested in how PC pumps (that's what we usually call these related squeeze exercises) benefit the male anatomy and sexual stamina.

Exercise: PC Flex

Your first sexual muscle exercise is the PC Flex. To do PC Flexes, you squeeze and release your PC muscle at the rate of your normal breathing. Hold it on the "in" breath and release it on the "out" breath, relaxing all your muscles as you do. Each cycle should take a few seconds. Start with 20 contractions, two or three times a day, and build up to at least 75 per set. When you feel you're good at this, switch to PC Clenches.

Exercise: PC Clench

Here's your second major exercise, PC Clenches. To do clenches, hold the squeeze for a longer period of time. Some experts say 6 seconds, some say 15, some say more. I suggest you start with 10-second cycles and slowly work up to longer ones, even minutes.

First, inhale and clench your PC, holding it tightly. Then push it out and relax for the same amount of time before your next clench. Repeat this cycle 20 times twice a day at first. As with flexes, build up to 75 reps twice a day.

The clench, contracting while inhaling and holding, is the skill you'll be using very soon to move sexual energy up out of your jewel region. This tool, which I call the PC Pump, is one of the keys to separating orgasm from ejaculation and having multiple orgasms.

Exercise: Devamani Elevations

Now for the weirdest-sounding of all the PC exercises: Devamani Elevations. Remember, devamani means divine jewels, so I use it here to mean testicles.

Yes, with enough dedicated practice, you can develop the muscle control to raise and lower your devamani on command.

Except for being just another peculiar way to strengthen and tone your PC, why should you care? You care because your devamani elevate before you can ejaculate. You can't fire a gun if the hammer isn't cocked, right? So if you have the mastery to lower your testicles consciously, you prevent or delay what used to seem inevitable.

Devamani Elevations take a much higher level of PC muscle mastery than the average guy has. So I recommend you don't put a lot of effort into them until you're real good at PC Clenches.

When you're ready for Devamani Elevations, here's how to practice:

Stand with your feet shoulder-width apart or sit on the edge of a bed or coffee table. In the sitting position, you can cup the bottom of your testicles or make a thumb-forefinger ring above them so you can feel them moving slightly.

Tighten your PC underneath your devamani and pull them in, holding for a few seconds. Then push them out for a few seconds. Relax for a moment before the next contraction. Begin by doing a couple of sets of 20 per day, working up to 75 each time. Devamani elevations may seem difficult at first, so you'll probably be using all of your PC, front and back, in addition to your abdominal muscles.

It's also interesting to practice with an erection. One expert even recommends practicing bouncing a towel.

A friend told me about one of his single male clients who was extremely popular in his social circle, especially with women. Actually, he had a real reputation for making love all night.

How did he develop that talent? Through some of the same study and exercises you're engaged in here, he learned that a man's devamani naturally pull in to the body just before ejaculation. This is probably a natural defense mechanism against getting kicked at just the wrong time. Anyway, this well-known stud worked his PC long and hard to the point where he could push his devamani away from his body when he got too close to 9.9. For some guys, that's enough to drop their arousal down to a manageable level.

This is an advanced technique, so please don't force yourself trying to make it work right now. One of my readers didn't listen to this advice and gave himself a groin strain that lasted for weeks by trying to go too fast. In a few weeks or months, maybe this will be a valuable tool for your sexual stamina. For now, just consider it a pep talk to get you motivated to do your exercises.

Guidelines for PC Exercises

I know you're a tough guy who can handle a little pain now and then. Unfortunately, pain won't help this program. Instead, use the easy-going approach and build up gradually.

Again, I want to remind you about the first R of RAMPER. That's relax, right? These exercises may be about squeezing your PC muscle, but the relaxing in between each contraction is vital.

If you're tense, your sexual energy gets trapped and can't flow. When it builds up in vajra, he does what he knows best to release it. Consequently, the unflexed moments between pumps are as important as the strengthening. Sure, get into the habit of squeezing to tone the muscles while doing your exercises, but put as much attention on relaxing totally between flexes.

That's why it's vital to relax everything else when you do PC pumps. During your first couple weeks, you may find that you're also tightening your stomach, butt, or leg muscles. Don't worry about it for now. Within a few days or weeks, you'll learn to isolate your muscle control so you'll only flex the pelvic floor where the PC resides.

You Need to Make This a Daily Regimen

Maybe the most important lesson about strengthening your sexual muscles is regularity. No, not going to the toilet regularly. Practicing your exercises regularly.

Doing PC pumps is easy. The hard part for most people is establishing a regimen that works, then remembering to do it. To get the maximum benefits from this program, I urge you to commit to making your PC exercises a part of your daily routine right away.

Develop some successful memory devices so that you don't forget. Find a few times and places where you'll remember to do several sets each day. If you can practice each exercise three or four times a day, it's even better, especially at the start. Just don't push it too fast and make yourself sore by straining your crotch at the outset. Once your pelvis gets strong (after several months of practice), you'll still need to continue your regimen as a maintenance program.

What kind of memory joggers do I recommend? You might use taking a shower, while you're commuting to and from work, stopping for traffic lights, sitting in boring meetings, checking your email, watching TV commercials, or when you start your workout at the gym.

I use some daily life rituals for my reminders—brushing my teeth, soaking in the hot tub, and taking our two frisky golden retrievers for daily walks. Chairlift rides during ski season work well for me, too, since I ski more than 40 days a winter. But I need more practice in the summer. Whatever you choose, do it regularly so it becomes an integral part of your life routine. Since it doesn't seem to matter—choose whenever and wherever best jogs your memory.

I've developed a powerful tool to get you off to a rousing start with your PC regimen. It's called my Tantric Sex Muscle

Ecourse. This ecourse is a series of seven short lessons that will teach you more exercises, give you more background, and, above all, remind you to practice at the outset. For more information visit www.tantraattahoe.com.

OPENING SENSES

Did anyone ever suggest to you that the way to avoid ejaculating was by thinking about baseball, work, or your grandmother? Well, this part of Male Multiple Orgasm is the exact opposite. It's about paying maximum attention to the sensations that arise in every part of your body. By opening your senses more, you can enjoy each little moment of pleasure to the fullest.

Use the Cornerstone of Presence

These next exercises are all about developing the A of RAMPER, namely awareness of your body. This is how you will learn to be more present and focus in the right direction. Do you remember that presence and visualization together are one of the four cornerstones of ecstatic sex?

Of course, this requires slowing down and relaxing into the experience. Your aim is to engage all of your erogenous zones and your whole body. When you relax into the feelings in your feet, butt, chest, and nipples (just to suggest a few subtle erogenous zones that may excite you), you shift your focus away from your jewels. This is a basic premise of Male Multiple Orgasm: spreading the energy away from your jewels, so you can have whole body orgasms without an immediate ejaculation.

I know that it's one thing to practice by yourself and another when you're with a wildly animated partner. But believe me, most lovers really want the slow, sensitive, savoring attention that opening your senses brings. Let's start solo anyway and worry about keeping up with your partner once you've mastered the basics.

Exercise: Walking Meditation

Walking Meditation is a sensory experience designed to open multiple senses at once. Practice this exercise in a safe place outside where you won't be interrupted (maybe your back yard when no one is home?), or inside if necessary. Take your shoes off if you're inside or if it's safe outside to walk barefoot where you practice. You can wear clothes for this exercise, but it's also great if you can do it in the nude, especially outside if you enjoy that.

1) Close your eyes and stand still comfortably, watching your breath for a few minutes until you feel relaxed.

2) Feel the level of tension and relaxation in every muscle starting with your feet and moving up to the top of your head.

3) Next, while maintaining total awareness of your body, walk very, very slowly with maximum consciousness. Don't open your eyes completely, but keep them softly focused so you don't hurt yourself. Move as slowly as you can, feeling the minute movements of every muscle as you lift each foot and leg. Feel the pressure and motion of your whole body as you set a foot down and shift your weight. Notice the texture of the grass or floor, or the hardness and level of the ground.

4) After a few minutes of complete focus on the physical sensations of walking, begin to pay attention to your sense of sight. As you open your eyes more, observe slowly and in detail what you see: shapes, textures, and colors. Continue to maintain total awareness of your body. If you accidentally shift your entire attention to your sense of sight as you're walking, remind yourself to keep feeling what's happening as well.

5) When you're ready for more, add your sense of hearing. Listen for any and all sounds around you. If you're outside, you might hear the wind, the rustle of leaves, birds, and cars. If you're inside, you might be amazed at all the ambient sounds all around you: creaking walls and floors,

plumbing and heating, and noises from computers and appliances. Now you're sensing your body, sight, and hearing all together.

6) Finally, add your sense of smell. If you're outside in the spring, there will be many wonderful scents on the wind. Whenever and wherever you are though, pay attention to anything your nose picks up.

I don't know a safe way by yourself to add the sense of taste outside, but it's something you can have a lot of fun with inside.

At some points in this exercise, you'll probably tune out and forget to focus on one or more senses. Unless you're a yoga master, expect it and don't worry. Just keep practicing every day or so until you can spread your attention throughout all the sensory input reaching you for a few moments. You'll be amazed how much this will increase your pleasure during lovemaking, whether solo or with a partner. And it's essential to be able to master your ejaculation response.

Exercise: Ejaculation Awareness

You now get to begin one of the most enjoyable parts of this program: self-pleasuring vajra. The first exercise is designed to heighten your awareness of your ejaculation response, the point of no return, emission, and expulsion. Actually, it belongs in the next section, but I've put a copy here in case you unexpectedly slip over the edge during the remaining exercises. That way you'll know how to take full advantage of this joyous experience and learn from it whenever it happens.

I'm not kidding about praising the very thing you're trying to control. Part of this exercise is to enjoy the intense pleasure of ejaculating. At the same time, you'll learn to recognize the energy and sensations you'll need to spread throughout your body to prolong lovemaking. So read this exercise now, use it if you slip, but otherwise wait until later to practice intentionally. OK, got it?

By the way, there's no penalty for doing this exercise multiple times, planned and unplanned. The more you learn about your body's responses, the better you'll be at Male Multiple Orgasm. As we discussed earlier, there's a price to learning how to play on the edge of ejaculation. The good news/bad news is that at times you'll stumble and let go, until you develop the knack of comfortably flirting with 9.9. Part of this exercise is to accept and enjoy the experience instead of dreading it.

1) Self-pleasure vajra slowly, feeling all your sensations fully.

2) As you reach the point of no return, stop all motion.

3) Relax by taking deep breaths and focus your attention on all parts of your body, especially your jewels.

4) As you start to ejaculate, feel the semen moving from your devamani (testicles) to the base of vajra with smooth muscle contractions (emission phase).

5) Notice the delay between phases and then the involuntary squeezes of your pelvic muscles as they cause the semen to squirt out (expulsion phase).

6) Now focus on what you learned and give thanks that you can experience such intense pleasure.

Exercise: Whole Body Sensory Focus

A general aim of Male Multiple Orgasm is to become more aware of your body and how you respond during sex, from initial excitement, through full arousal, to the time you reach orgasm. In this exercise, you'll use gentle self-massage all over your body to achieve this exploration.

1) Sit or lie down nude in a relaxed posture in a safe, comfortable, uninterrupted space.

2) Take a few deep belly breaths to relax and let go of any stress you've been carrying.

3) Using one hand at first, lightly and slowly touch your whole body, excluding your jewels. You want to use what some call a "taking touch"—which means to feel as much

with the touching hand as with the part that's being caressed.

4) Explore all parts of your body gently and slowly, except your jewels, as if you were a young child with a new toy. Experiment with different strokes on different body parts, feeling each sensation as if for the first time.

5) You're still breathing deeply and slowly in your belly, right?

6) Next, do the same with your jewels, vajra (penis) as well as your devamani (testicles) and anywhere around there that turns you on. Explore your favorite parts in the same child-like way, lightly and slowly, without trying to make yourself explode. (We'll get to that part of the exercise later.) By the way, if you do go past the point of no return, enjoy it. If it takes you awhile to recharge your sensitivity, you might want to take a break before resuming this exercise.

7) Next, include your whole body in the same way, excluding nothing.

8) If this turns you on and you get hard, well, that's great! Feel those excited feelings fully. How does being turned-on affect different parts of your body: hair, nipples, devamani, vajra, etc? Sense how all the parts of your body feel different to the hands taking touch when you're excited?

Exercise: Self-Pleasuring Discovery

Male Multiple Orgasm is about increasing pleasure of all kinds. The spiritual attitude that's the foundation of this program is to honor, almost worship, pleasure as a divine gift. That's why you won't ever find me using the term masturbation, since that's got all kinds of hidden, guilty, dirty connotations.

This exercise is about self-pleasuring, giving yourself the gift of the maximum enjoyment your body affords. OK, it still means playing with your jewels, but you're supposed to do it with an open, accepting, and appreciating attitude.

Since this is an appreciation exercise, you don't need to use lubrication (such as petroleum jelly), which increases sensitivity. If you're really sensitive, you'll probably want to do Self-Pleasuring Discovery dry at this point. Later, you can use some kind of self-pleasuring cream. But as with everything in this program, it's up to you.

When you're ready, you'll want to use an oil-based lubricant to heighten the stimulation. There are lots of options at sex shops. Many people use massage oil or baby oil. My favorite is Albolene, a make-up remover you can get at big drugstores. If you prefer completely natural things, try olive oil. Your partner may prefer water-based lubricants during sexual union. These work well at first for self-pleasuring until they dry out, which is quickly. Though you can use a spray bottle filled with water to recharge it, it's more complicated than something that stays slippery all by itself.

1) Find a comfortable, safe, uninterrupted place to practice in the nude. Some people enjoy self-pleasuring rituals. Try sitting on the floor cross-legged in meditation position in front of a full-length mirror, with candles burning and sensual music playing.

2) While observing your body from above or in a mirror, begin deep slow belly breathing to relax and charge your energy system.

3) Start pleasuring yourself wherever feels good. Experiment to find what arousal pattern works best for you.

4) When you begin stroking vajra, remember to go slowly, relax, and enjoy. Open all your senses, continuing deep belly breathing. Don't be in a hurry! Give yourself those wonderful turned-on feelings, and experience each sensation fully.

5) Experiment with different strokes, speeds, and pressures to find out what creates which sensations and what's most intensely pleasurable. Here are some things to try:

- Alternate hands to see which feels better.
- Try up-strokes, down-strokes, thumb forward, and thumb back.
- Concentrate on vajra's shaft, on the head (glans or crown), and the frenulum (the sensitive underside of the head).
- Use your thumb and forefinger as a ring upward and downward with thumb forward and back.
- Roll vajra between both hands like a rolling pin, and use both hands from mid-shaft out or from top and bottom to middle.
- Rub vajra's underside with the flat of your hand, and press or roll vajra against your belly or thigh.
- Pull or tickle your devamani with the other hand.
- Use the corkscrew, rotating your hand as it slides up, and the pop-off, squeezing while you suddenly pull your hand up and over vajra's head.

Some of these may be rough or uncomfortable without lubrication. If you find that to be the case, do the comfortable ones first and then use an oil or cream for the others.

6) And don't forget the rest of your body. Remember to use your other hand to arouse your nipples, devamani, pubic bone, perineum (between your anus and devamani), and anus. Nothing is off-limits if it turns you on. Again, your aim is to feel more, not to ejaculate. But if you do, well, great! Just come back and finish the exercise when you're ready.

Now wasn't that fun? Did you learn anything new? If not, did you at least relax and enjoy yourself?

Exercise: Self-Pleasuring Vocally

Sound is one of the Four Cornerstones of sexual ecstasy. Because most of us are conditioned to be quiet during sex, few realize the potential power of sound to stimulate and regulate excitement. Using the sounds that naturally emanate from your body when it's feeling pleasure is a great way to circulate energy and spread the urge to ejaculate. This exercise is the same as the previous one with one change: you get to verbalize.

Some people find this difficult at first, because it's so different from what they're accustomed to doing. But then you've already accepted the idea that you need to change dramatically to be a Master of Orgasms, right? Besides, most lovers really love an expressive, passionate partner in the sack. Here's a great way to reinforce your commitment to transform your sexuality:

1) Find a practice space where there's no chance of being overheard. If you live within thin walls, have roommates, or close neighbors, this might mean a hike into the wilderness for practicing.

2) Repeat the Self-Pleasuring Discovery Exercise, concentrating on your favorite moves. These are the things you learned that give you the greatest pleasure.

3) Feel what you are doing and allow each sensation to become its own sound. Use moans, groans, grunts, growls, cries, sighs, whines, or even laughs. To emphasize your earthy nature, visualize animals and make the kind of sounds they make.

4) One at a time, practice using the vowels: A, E, I, O, U. Some work great for expressing different pleasurable feelings.

5) Once you get accustomed to converting feeling into sounds, practice making your verbalizations twice as loud. You may have to force it at first, but give it a try. Then double the volume again and again until you're screaming.

6) You're probably still breathing deeply, because you can't be vocal without breath. Visualize the breath going into your erogenous zones, fueling the pleasure you're creating. And then visualize the sound moving that excited sexual energy up, around, and out.

Does it make sense when I say these exercises are cumulative? What I mean is that each little skill adds up to Orgasm Mastery. So you should naturally be incorporating everything you learn into later exercises. From here on out you're going to relax, breathe slowly and deeply in the belly, keep all your senses open, make sounds that express how you're feeling, and enjoy yourself at all times. You're doing all that now, right? If not, practice this exercise some more and be sure you follow these guidelines from now on.

How many times and how long you do each exercise depends, for the most part, on you. Part of Male Multiple Orgasm is developing your own judgment about how you're doing and what warrants more practice. You may want to repeat some of these exercises frequently or routinely. Keep doing the ones that make you feel good. From here on, if you find you're not relaxed or you can't focus all your senses during an upcoming practice, go back and continue the relaxing and opening exercises discussed earlier in this chapter.

MEASURED SELF-PLEASURING: USING THE 10-POINT AROUSAL LEVEL SCALE

Now, we're going to add the M—measuring your arousal level—to the relaxation and awareness you're developing (see page 36 for my 10-point scale for monitoring your excitement level). Here's where we start using this scale intensively. As you practice the following self-pleasuring exercises (and later with a partner), continually monitor your position on the scale. But your definitions will probably be somewhat different than mine. You'll undoubtedly find sensations and signals that will work better for you to define each level. Gradually, you'll make up your own scale.

Exercise: Ejaculation Awareness

Whether you've ejaculated during the previous sensual exercises or not, it's time to consciously practice feeling as much as you can when you have a wet orgasm. This is a repeat of what I included in the previous section, but at this point you're supposed to master it. The exercise is simple: get yourself off and enjoy it.

Since Ejaculation Awareness is designed to increase your consciousness of the physical changes your body experiences during explosive orgasm, you should do this as slowly as you can. Have you ever tried to make it last as long as possible? Well, now you will. Imagine you're a witness to a scientific experiment. Your assignment is to mentally record the input you receive from all your senses. That's why you spent that time practicing open senses.

1) Self-pleasure slowly, feeling all your sensations fully. Use lubricant to heighten your sensitivity if you want.

2) As you use different strokes to turn yourself on, simply notice your level of arousal rising on the 10-point scale. Your definitions will probably evolve to be different than mine.

3) Are you aware of changes in your body? Heart rate, muscle tension, breathing, tight devamani, etc.?

4) When you reach 9.9, the point of no return, stop all motion.

5) Relax by taking deep breaths and focus your attention on all parts of your body, especially your jewels.

6) As you ejaculate, feel the semen moving from your devamani to the base of vajra with smooth muscle contractions (emission phase).

7) Notice the delay between phases and then the involuntary squeezes of your pelvic PC muscles as they cause the collected semen to squirt out (expulsion phase).

8) Now focus on what you learned and give thanks that you can experience such intense pleasure.

Did you notice the changes your body experienced as you got close to 9.9? Could you feel the point of no return and the internal emission contractions of your prostate before the expulsion caused by your pelvic muscles? If not, why don't you try it again when you're ready. Repeat the exercise until you can really feel what's happening down there.

Exercise: Self-Pleasuring by the Numbers

A major part of self-monitoring during your individual practices will be learning how close you can go to 9.9 without slipping over the edge. Up to this point, we haven't made a big deal about avoiding ejaculation or regulating how excited you are.

Now, to develop greater awareness and mastery over your orgasms, we're going to repeat the previous exercise with a numerical twist. Hopefully, you've been noticing your level of arousal at each moment during the previous exercises. Now, Self-Pleasuring by the Numbers asks you to excite yourself to a specific level and then stop. Of course, we'll be upping the ante at each step, getting closer and closer to the top. Maybe you'll go over the top and maybe you won't. For our purposes here, it doesn't matter much, as long as you're tuning in to your level of arousal.

1) Self-pleasure slowly, feeling all your sensations fully. Use lubricant to heighten your sensitivity if you want.

2) When your arousal level reaches 4, stop all motion, relax everywhere including your pelvis by taking deep breaths, focus your attention on your entire body, especially your jewels, and drink in the pleasure.

3) When your excitement drops to 2, start self-pleasuring again. This could be a few seconds or a few minutes.

4) When you reach 6 on the scale, stop, relax, breathe, and enjoy.

5) When your excitement drops to 2 again, begin again.

6) When you reach 8, stop, relax, breathe, and enjoy.

7) When your excitement drops to 2 again, begin again.

8) When you reach 9, stop, relax, breathe, and enjoy.

9) If you choose, repeat this cycle over and over, pausing at each point on the scale (3, 4, 5, etc.) and seeing how close you can skirt 9.9 without ejaculating.

Actually, that's all there is to the M of RAMPER. You'll probably want to repeat this practice until you're really clear on your own definition of each of the numbers. Make up your own definitions if that helps you identify the excitement at each level.

That's Enough Solo Prep

Well, that wraps up the Solo Prep Chapter. You've learned to relax, be more sensitive, breathe, make sounds, feel things, and measure your turn-on. You've started to regularly strengthen your sexual muscles, right?

You could spend a few months really perfecting all these foundations of Orgasm Mastery. Hopefully, you've at least spent some weeks getting to where you can apply these fundamental skills automatically. Next, we'll employ these exact tools to stretch the time you can maintain excitement and learn to savor pleasure without worrying too much about falling over the cliff.

If you have an intimate partner and haven't done it already, it's time to report in. Briefly explain what you've practiced, how it's made you feel, and how you expect it will ultimately change your lovemaking.

CHAPTER 5

✧ *Solo Mastery*

With the basic exercises well-practiced, you're ready for Solo Mastery. This chapter is about learning to stay at the point of no return indefinitely. Interested? I bet!

Chapter 5 begins by teaching peaking: how to go from 1 on the 10-point arousal scale up to 9 or so and back down again quickly while self-pleasuring. The second section is a series of both modern and ancient physical techniques to interrupt ejaculation when you get too close. That's followed by a series of exercises that teach Orgasmic Breathing, a method of using the Four Cornerstones to stimulate and stabilize your pleasure. Finally, the rest of this chapter presents plateauing, how to maintain a high level of arousal while continuing stimulation.

As you might expect, this chapter is primarily concerned with the Ps of RAMPER—pacing, peaking, and plateauing. Though they belong more to E (energy circulation), I've thrown in some breathing exercises before plateauing. Because the breath is so vital in channeling sexual energy away from your jewels, it really is fundamental to learning to float in the plateau of ecstasy for long periods of time. The sooner you incorporate that into your practice, the better.

Though I won't repeat it each time, I'm reminding you now to always set up a safe, comfortable, uninterrupted space for practice, use appropriate background music, relax, clear your mind, and breathe first. You'll remember, won't you?

CLIMBING UP AND DOWN THE PEAKS

Peaking is all about letting your excitement rise to a high level and then immediately drop back down. Do you remember the graph of your arousal that appears on page 38? The line that demonstrates peaking looks like a mountain climber scaling a steep mountain, going up sharply and then precipitously back down.

I'm going to show you a bunch of ways to rapidly reduce your excitement. Obviously, both relaxation and finely-tuned senses are essential to learning peaking. Breath will play a big part, too. We'll begin with stopping stimulation altogether just before 9.9. Then you'll learn how to do reduce vajra's excitement level using subtle changes in how you're stimulating yourself.

Exercise: Stop-Start Peaking

In Stop-Start Peaking, you'll practice extending the time you can stimulate yourself without ejaculating. This exercise will be familiar because it begins just like Self-Pleasuring by the Numbers, which you did in the last chapter. At first, aim to stay hard without letting go during a 15-minute practice. Then work up to 30 minutes of self-pleasure without ejaculating during repeated exercises. Experts say if you can continue to self-pleasure for 30 minutes without losing it, you can maintain it for much longer. No matter how sensitive you are, this is possible through practice.

1) Self-pleasure vajra with a dry hand until you reach an arousal level of 6.

2) Immediately stop all stimulation, open your eyes wide, relax all your muscles, take deep slow breaths, and wait until your excitement drops to a level 4.

3) Repeat steps 1 and 2 five more times. Note how later cycles differ from the first one or two.

4) Continue the exercise by repeating these steps up to an arousal level of 8. When you reach the peak, wait until you've dropped to 6 before continuing.

5) Continue the exercise by repeating these steps up to an arousal level of 9. When you reach the peak, wait until you've dropped to 7 before continuing.

6) Now extend your pleasure stamina by repeatedly stopping and starting. Again and again, pleasure vajra up to arousal level 9 and then stop for a moment before continuing.

7) Remember, if you slip over the edge and ejaculate, relax and enjoy it. It's good news that you're pushing your limits. You might have to practice many times to develop the sensitivity and timing that you want. But you can do it! OK, now that my pep talk is over, pick up the exercise where you left off. You'll probably be less excitable after a little release, so developing the stop-start reflexes should be easier.

8) When you can maintain self-pleasuring for 30 minutes by stopping and starting without ejaculating, repeat steps 1 through 6 using a lubricated hand. (If you don't have a favorite self-pleasuring cream, refer to the suggestions about lubrication in the Resources section at the back of the book.

Stop-Start Peaking simulates what you'll be doing soon with a partner. Keep practicing to stretch the time you can enjoy pleasure longer and longer without exploding. Once you get the hang of it, you may want to practice getting closer and closer to arousal level 9.9. Enjoy a long pleasurable session up to and back down from the low 9s. Then push it, knowing you will eventually finish with a satisfying wet orgasm. Treat it as your reward for a job well done.

When you can pleasure vajra to high peaks of arousal with lubrication for 30 minutes or more, move on to the next exercise.

Exercise: Subtle Adjustments Peaking

Hopefully, you've practiced Stop-Start Peaking enough that you've developed the confidence to back off when you need to.

But what if you're with a partner who is so excited that you don't want to interrupt the flow? That's where Subtle Adjustments Peaking can help. In Subtle Adjustments Peaking, you'll repeat the previous exercise, except you'll make small changes in how you're pleasuring vajra, instead of stopping entirely. Sometimes, missing a stroke, slowing a bit, or gliding up and down vajra less firmly will allow you to maintain your arousal level when you're making love.

1) Self-pleasure vajra slowly up to arousal level 6 with a dry hand.

2) Instead of stopping stimulation, vary what you're doing to reduce the excitement a few points (for example, from arousal level 6 down to 4). Slow down, lighten the pressure of your strokes, or change direction. If you're on vajra's head, move to the shaft. If you've been enjoying long strokes, shorten them.

3) Follow the same regimen as Stop-Start Peaking, repeating each series six times up to arousal levels 6, 8, and 9, or more.

4) Now extend your pleasure stamina using subtle adjustments. Again and again, pleasure vajra up to arousal level 9 and then interrupt the ascent for a moment before continuing.

5) When you can continue pleasuring vajra for 30 minutes using subtle adjustments to drop your excitement level a few points, repeat the whole process with a lubricated hand.

Subtle Adjustments Peaking will come in handy soon since you'll use it during sexual union later in the program. Is it obvious how critical these last two exercises are? Master them completely through repetition before moving on. When you can get to arousal level 9 and back off without stopping or ejaculating for 30 minutes, you're ready to include the energy techniques that follow. But before you do, take a moment to appreciate your progress. By learning to pace yourself up to this point, you've transformed your sexual pattern into one that already closely resembles the lovemaking reality you want to create.

Exercise: Breath Peaking

Ultimately, Male Multiple Orgasm is an energetic process in which you bask at high states of arousal, circulating orgasmic energy throughout your body and exchanging it with a partner. That's why I recommend you start practicing the energy-oriented version of peaking here. Breath Peaking is one of the key subtle methods of pacing yourself and reducing your excitement during lovemaking. Since we all tend to breathe through the mouth during orgasm, you're going to switch to nasal breathing here because it's less arousing.

1) Self-pleasure vajra slowly up to arousal level 6 with either a dry or lubricated hand, depending on how sensitive you feel and how well you've done with previous mastery exercises.

2) Slow your rate of breathing.

3) Open your eyes wide and inhale more deeply into your belly, breathing through your NOSE and holding your breath for a moment. Don't stop stimulating vajra, but slow down slightly if you need to at first while you're learning.

4) Relax completely as you exhale, visualizing your sexual fire streaming out of vajra. Moan with pleasure to release energy.

5) Inhale again through the nose, visualizing energy moving up vajra through your pelvis to your heart or even higher.

6) Can you feel your excitement lessen simply by slowing your breath? Play with it until you can, using stop-start and subtle adjustments as needed.

7) Follow the same regimen as with the peaking exercises, repeating each series six times up to arousal levels 6, 8, and 9, or higher.

8) Fast panting releases energy suddenly for some guys. Try it.

9) As you practice getting closer and closer to ejaculation, see if you can back your excitement off and pace yourself just by slowing and deepening your breath through the nose.

INTERRUPTING EJACULATION

In this section, I've collected both ancient and modern techniques that you can use to interrupt ejaculation when you get too close to arousal level 9.9. I've included this in the spirit of completeness, knowing some things work better for some guys than others.

Actually, these exercises are a bit of a departure from the program you're on. They're really stopgaps if you feel yourself slipping over the edge. You see, by practicing interrupting ejaculation, we're back on the "control" wagon, trying to stop the energy that's flowing. As I hope you're grasping, Male Multiple Orgasm is about flowing with the rising energy, channeling it, and enjoying it. It's about putting yourself in a position where you don't have to concentrate on stopping anything.

That said, I want you to try all of the exercises mentioned in this section. All you've got to waste is a little sperm, right? These methods really are different versions of the stop-and-start method we did in the peaking section. I'm hoping that one or more will work really well for you, so you can add it to your arsenal of lovemaking tools. I've presented them as separate exercises, but feel free to try several of them at once if that works better for you.

Yippee, You've Got a G-Spot, Too

Do you remember your perineum, the part of your pelvic floor between your devamani and rosetta (anus)? Below the base of vajra, there's a soft spot through which you can apply pressure to your prostate that's called your Perineum Point. Some prefer to call it the Prostate Point, and, because it's so valuable, some call it the Million Dollar Point.

If you don't know where your perineum is, take a little break now and search for the little indentation down there that has less resistance to pushing in and up. It should feel good deep inside when you find it and press hard.

The prostate is the male equivalent of a woman's G-Spot. Have you ever had an erotic prostate massage either externally or through your rosetta? Though the internal variety takes some hygiene precautions like immediate finger disinfecting or use of rubber gloves, the pleasure it gives can be incredible once learned. By the way, I'm in no way talking about those insensitive exams doctors give, shoving their finger up your anus to check the size of your prostate.

Occasional firm rhythmic pulsing pressure on your Perineum Point can be highly pleasurable if applied with skill and sensitivity. Stroking vajra and your G-Spot at the same time can be incredible, lengthening and intensifying all kinds of orgasms, especially the explosive ones. In fact, the male G-Spot is what we call the "sacred gate" to multiple orgasm for men. It's such a big and unexplored subject that I wrote a book about it. Look in the Resources section at the back of *Male Multiple Orgasm* for more information.

Exercise: Perineum Press

Some say prostate massage is good for your health, but our main concern here is how to interrupt ejaculation. Fortunately, it helps with that, too. For many men, prostate stimulation reduces the likelihood of exploding involuntarily since it purges the gland of the fluid necessary for emission. If you push hard on your Perineum Point right before the point of no return, it blocks the emission phase. The Perineum Press prevents seminal fluid from entering the urethral canal when the spasms start.

Even if you have orgasmic contractions, the semen remains and is reabsorbed. This is a great way to experience dry orgasm, pleasurable contractions without ejaculating. But look out, if you stimulate your prostate, your anus, the buried base of vajra, or your devamani too late, it can push you over the edge to ejaculation.

1) Self-pleasure vajra using a dry or lubricated hand as you prefer.

2) When you reach arousal level 6, stop all motion, locate your Perineum Point, and press upward firmly in one steady motion for 10 to 30 seconds or until you drop down a few arousal points.

3) When your excitement drops, continue self-pleasuring up to arousal level 8, stop, and press again.

4) Repeat the exercise up to arousal level 8 again. This time, however, see if you can continue stroking while pressing on your Perineum Point and having your arousal drop.

5) Keep practicing the exercise using the Perineum Press, seeing how close you can get to arousal level 9.9 and still back off.

6) If you haven't slipped over the edge and ejaculated yet, pleasure yourself up to 9.9 and see if you can interrupt the emission phase just before it starts by using the Perineum Press.

With a little luck and repeated practice, you should be able to experience dry orgasms with this technique. But never fear if the knack eludes you. The energy exercises you'll learn later are highly effective in teaching men to experience multiple orgasms.

Exercise: PC Squeeze

Once you've strengthened your PC muscle through several weeks of exercise, you'll have a more convenient way of interrupting ejaculation. Tightening your PC firmly has the same effect on your prostate as the Perineum Press. It's like putting on the car brakes when you find yourself on the verge of sliding over one of those really steep San Francisco streets. When you master PC Squeezes, you'll have another method, a very pleasurable one, to peak your excitement level. And it's less obtrusive to use while you're making love.

1) To warm up before stimulating vajra, do 30 PC Pumps to tone your muscles and massage your prostate. (Some

believe this internal massage all by itself can delay ejaculatory spasms from sweeping over you quickly.)

2) Self-pleasure vajra using a dry or lubricated hand as you prefer.

3) When you reach arousal level 6, stop all motion, hold your breath with your eyes wide open, and clamp down as tight as you can on your PC muscle until your arousal subsides several points.

4) Stimulate yourself again up to arousal level 6, but this time pump your PC repeatedly while you continue stroking. Do these pumps excite you more, or do they spread the energy? This experiment will help you choose your preferred PC pumping technique.

5) Repeat the self-pleasuring, continuing this time until you reach arousal level 8. Use one long hard squeeze, two medium squeezes, or several quick PC squeezes— whichever works best for you to reduce your excitement.

6) Keep practicing the exercise using the PC Squeeze, seeing how close you can get to 9.9 and still back off.

7) If you haven't slipped over the edge yet, pleasure yourself up to arousal level 9.9 and see if you can interrupt the emission phase just before it starts by using the PC Squeeze.

If you're not eminently successful with PC Squeezes right off the bat, please don't get discouraged. This takes savvy timing as well as more strength than most guys realize at first. So if you're struggling with this technique, don't despair. Use your frustration to fuel your more regular and intense PC exercises.

Exercise: Root Lock

One branch of Chinese Taoism offers many methods of spiritual and energetic sexuality, which are similar to Tantra and Yoga. A powerful Taoist and Yoga technique is the Root Lock, which resembles the PC Squeeze in some ways.

To perform a Root Lock, hold your breath momentarily and push your pelvic muscles out as though you were straining to empty your bowels. Ancient Tibetans called it "closing the lower gate." They advise you to tighten your rosetta, turn your tongue and eyes upward, contract the joints of your feet and hands, tighten your fingers, and pull in your stomach to the backbone. Yoga adds that while expelling the breath through your nose, contract your anal muscles, drawing them inward and upward. They all work together, except some say push out and others say pull in. Let's try it both ways:

1) Self-pleasure vajra using a dry or lubricated hand as you prefer.

2) When you reach arousal level 6, stop all motion and do a Root Lock. Expel all your breath and hold it, keep your eyes wide open looking upward, push your tongue on the roof of your mouth, tighten your fingers, hands, and feet, and push out on your rosetta until your arousal subsides several points.

3) Stimulate yourself again up to arousal level 6, do another Root Lock, but this time contract your anal muscles inward and upward while pulling your stomach toward your spine. Which works better for you, in or out?

4) Repeat the self-pleasuring, continuing this time until you reach arousal level 8, and then do your preferred Root Lock.

5) Keep practicing the exercise using Root Locks, seeing how close you can get to 9.9 and still back off.

6) If you haven't slipped over the edge yet, pleasure yourself up to arousal level 9.9 and see if you can interrupt the emission phase of ejaculation just before it starts by using the Root Lock.

Exercise: Vajra Squeeze

Knowing what causes hard-ons—blood flowing into vajra—gives you the power to stop them. If you squeeze in the right place, you can force blood out of vajra and reduce your erection. This helps many men delay their explosive orgasms.

If you do a Vajra Squeeze just before the point of climax, experts report that you can essentially cancel the impending release. Some recommend vajra's tip, some the middle, and others the base. Again, I think it's worthwhile to practice everything to see what works best for you. Of course, squeezing the base is a lot more practical when making love.

1) Self-pleasure vajra using a dry or lubricated hand as you prefer.

2) When you reach arousal level 6, stop all motion and squeeze your FRENULUM behind vajra's crown and under his head. You can use your thumb on top and forefinger below or any other way that's convenient. Hold it for 10 to 30 seconds, or until the urge subsides.

3) Stimulate yourself again up to arousal level 6, this time squeezing the MIDDLE of vajra with your thumb and index finger until your arousal subsides several points.

4) Stimulate yourself again up to 6, this time squeezing the TIP of vajra with your thumb and index finger. Note which motion works better for you.

5) Repeat the self-pleasuring, continuing this time until you reach arousal level 8, and then do your preferred method of Vajra Squeeze.

6) Keep practicing the exercise using Vajra Squeezes, seeing how close you can get to arousal level 9.9 and still back off.

7) If you haven't slipped past the point of no return yet, pleasure yourself up to 9.9 and see if you can interrupt the emission phase just before it starts by using a Vajra Squeeze.

Exercise: Devamani Pull

When you ejaculate, your devamani (testicles) elevate or move up close to your body as your scrotum tightens. I've read that this is a built-in protection mechanism, and applies pressure to the sperm reservoir that responds to the contractions around the prostate. What do you think would happen if your testicles didn't elevate? Right, you wouldn't ejaculate. That's the theory of the Devamani Pull.

1) Self-pleasure vajra using a dry or lubricated hand as you prefer.

2) When you reach arousal level 6, stop all motion and hold vajra in one hand. With the other hand, make a ring with your thumb and forefinger above your devamani and pull down firmly. Be careful not to squeeze your testicles. Wait until your arousal subsides, which can take from 10 to 30 seconds.

3) Stimulate yourself again up to arousal level 6, this time grasping your scrotum between your devamani with your thumb and forefinger and pulling down firmly. Does this work better than the ring method?

4) Self-pleasure again up to arousal level 6. When you stop this time, see if you can consciously relax your body (like you learned in the PC Exercise section). Can you reduce your excitement level purely with muscle control this way?

5) Repeat the self-pleasuring, continuing this time until you reach arousal level 8, and then do your preferred method of Devamani Pull.

6) Keep practicing the exercise using Devamani Pulls, seeing how close you can get to 9.9 and still back off.

7) If you haven't slipped over the edge and ejaculated yet, pleasure yourself up to 9.9 and see if you can interrupt the emission phase just before it starts by using a Devamani Pull.

Many Taoist techniques are based on Chinese medicine, which works with energy as does acupuncture. Proponents of these techniques claim that you can avoid ejaculation by closing your mouth, rolling your eyes left and right, holding your breath, gnashing your teeth, moving your hands up and down, and pressing the Ping-I acupoint one inch above the right nipple with the index and middle finger of the left hand.

The *Kama Sutra*, the famous Indian love guide, also suggests a potent retention technique in which your partner slaps your butt and chest with an open palm. This is a hard one to practice on yourself, but give it a try if you want.

Hopefully, with all this stroking, you've found some methods that you can use in emergency situations. If not, I hope you've had lots of fun and fine-tuned your awareness of your arousal levels. Anyway, if you ask me, the following energy-related practices are much more powerful and useful.

ORGASMIC BREATHING

This section teaches you to combine many things you already know how to do in a way that propels the movement of orgasmic energy in your body. We're solidly in the E camp of RAMPER now, the realm of energy circulation.

Time to Master Subtle Orgasmic Energy

Orgasmic Breathing employs the kind of breath, sound, movement, and mental focus that happens when the average person has a typical exciting explosive orgasm. We're going to turn these components of the Four Cornerstones into tools you can use when you need to spread energy.

Here in the Solo Mastery Chapter, you're going to practice without sex for the most part so you can develop mastery over those body/mind functions that happen involuntarily during a climax. When you can use them to turn yourself on, you can use them to turn yourself off, too. Doesn't that make sense?

For the most part, we'll be dealing here with subtle energies. At first, don't expect that you'll be flipping one of those big high-voltage control levers with huge sparks that will throw your body across the room. Right away, if you're very relaxed and sensitive, or soon, hopefully, through practice, you'll become aware of a little warmth, electrical tingle, or pleasurable tickle.

It's like learning to tune in to a much higher-frequency sound than you're accustomed to. You've got to clear your mind and listen acutely to reach it. Once you learn to tune your receiver to subtle sexual energy, it becomes a powerful orgasmic force. You can direct and regulate it for magnified passion, lighting a slow burn instead of an overwhelming eruption.

Understand Why Tension Is Your Enemy

Can you understand how any mental or physical tension can prevent you from making progress at this stage? I bet, if you wanted to, that you could push your way through solid obstacles with your masculine force of will. Unfortunately, then you'd be working at cross-purposes to our goal here. You have to relax, breathe, and feel every little sensation to use subtle orgasmic energy. Otherwise, tension will block the doorway to feeling and moving these energies.

If, instead, you relax, don't worry about how fast you go, and never despair when it takes longer than you think it should, you'll soon get inklings, then surges, and finally waves that will bowl you over. But be patient. You'll probably need to practice numerous times for several weeks before the magic will occur.

Orgasmic Breathing may not appear to be directly dealing with vajra and his quickness on the draw. But it's an essential part of this program. The success of RAMPER depends on your ability to distribute the intense sexual energy that naturally collects in vajra throughout your body. When you simulate the physical and mental conditions of orgasm through this practice, you'll really have a leg up on ejaculation mastery.

Exercise: Breathing & Pumping

You know how to breathe properly and pump your PC already. Now we're going to combine these tools. At first, you'll want to do all these energy exercises naked or with loose clothing. Find a quiet space where you won't be interrupted. Play some suitable slow, sensuous, rhythmic music. Any slow hypnotic instrumental that turns you on will work fine.

1) Do this exercise lying down, standing with loose knees, sitting on the edge of a chair, or cross-legged on a pillow. Our favorite teaching position is on a *zafu*, a Japanese meditation pillow that's round, solid, and flattened top and bottom. If you can imagine squashing a ball of hamburger meat with your palm, you'll recognize a zafu when you see it.

2) Start with deep belly breathing. Close your eyes and breathe deeply and slowly in your belly. The more air you take in rhythmically, the more energy you'll be generating. I find it helps to pucker my mouth on the in-breath so I can hear the air rushing in. The complete Tantric breath has four stages: in, pause, out, pause. Pause for a distinct moment between inhaling and exhaling, and exhaling and inhaling.

3) After a few minutes of feeling cleansed, relaxed, and refreshed through breathing, begin clenching your PC on your inhale. Relax your PC along with everything else as you exhale.

4) Do you feel any sensations by breathing and pumping together? In your vajra, devamani, or elsewhere? Tune in and see if there are any subtle signals. Your first inklings may only be a little warmth, a whisper, or a tickle.

5) Once you've coordinated breathing and pumping, begin making sounds on your exhale. You can simply say "ahhh" as you let the air escape. Or you can use the other vowels ("eeee," "iiii," "oh," "oooo") to express any sensations you're feeling. If this is still awkward, push yourself to be louder and louder for a while. Then, when you lower the volume, it will feel more comfortable.

Exercise: Visualizing Energy

Next, we're going to add the visualization of energy along with your breathing and pumping. Since energy flows where attention goes, even if you just imagine sexual juice and electricity somewhere in your body, something will eventually happen. You already knew that the mind was the biggest sex organ, right? So I suggest you utilize it as much as possible, focusing your big head where it belongs, on creating pleasure.

We're going to begin working with your chakras (energy centers) in a big way. These are the vortices where energy tends to collect and swirl around at different places inside your body. For the common definitions of the seven chakras, see page 28.

Your inner flute is the invisible energy channel near your spine that connects your chakras. The visualizations of this exercise will begin opening that subtle conduit and flowing energy between the chakras.

1) Assume a similar comfortable position as in the previous exercise. Upright is probably better for visualizing rising and falling subtle energy.

2) Begin Breathing and Pumping again with eyes closed until you settle into a rhythm.

3) Rest one hand gently on your jewels, as if cradling a precious thing. This isn't designed for self-pleasuring, just as an anchor for moving energy. But if it turns you on, so much the better.

4) As you breathe in slowly, visualize the air entering through your first chakra at the base of your pelvis. As you breathe, use your other hand on your skin or floating just above your body to trace the energy flow you're visualizing in your mind's eye. After you move you hand gently up from your jewels to your belly as you breathe in, reverse it downward on your out-breath. Though your eyes are closed to contain your energy inside, look downward as you do this. Imagine the air is a fiery red stream of orgasmic energy.

5) After holding your breath for 10 seconds or so, exhale as you visualize the stream of energy flowing out through your first chakra. Relax completely for a moment before your next breath. Repeat this cycle several times.

6) Now on your in-breath, visualize the energy entering your first chakra and moving up your inner flute into your second chakra, your belly. As before, focus your eyes internally where you're visualizing, hold your breath, and exhale down your inner flute and out the first chakra. Repeat this a few times.

7) Repeat the sequence a few times each, moving energy from your first to your third through seventh chakras. In other words, imagine your breath moving from the first to the third, then the first to the fourth, and so on. In each case, picture the energy flowing from the first chakra to the upper chakra through your inner flute.

8) During this process, imagine that you're experiencing intensely passionate lovemaking, making your body move, your pulse quicken, and your sounds emanate from deep inside your reservoir of life force. And remember to keep all your senses open. If you feel any sensations, no matter how subtle, visualize your breath passing through where you feel them. In this way, the breath acts like adding fuel to a small fire, making it flare up. Even if you don't feel much, imagine that you do and breathe into the body parts you want to energize.

Exercise: Pelvic Rocking

One of the key Four Cornerstones is movement. PC pumps are powerful internal motions, but you need to include the rest of your body. If you've ever experienced a full-body orgasm where you writhe, undulate, and vibrate all over, you'll know what I mean. And if you haven't, boy, have you got something to look forward to.

Pelvic Rocking is a front-to-back and back-to-front rotation of your pelvic area. Some have likened it to riding a horse, but I prefer to compare it to slow, deep lovemaking when you're on top. With your weight on your knees and hands, the only way you can penetrate deeply is by either doing push-ups or by rocking your pelvis forward and backward. The latter is what we're adding to your repertoire here.

You might want to practice slow pelvic rocking with some primitive music like drums or African rhythms.

1) To get the feel of Pelvic Rocking, first try bouncing. Lie on your stomach and raise your hips up and down quickly. About the only way to do this is by rotating your hips. Then lie on your back. Put your feet flat on the floor with your knees bent, and roll your pelvis toward your feet and toward your head. That's the motion we're aiming for.

2) Kneel on your knees on a *zafu* turned on its side between your legs, with your feet behind you Japanese style. If you don't have one and can't make the position work with pillows, you can try it standing, lying down, or on the edge of a chair. Unfortunately, if you have to use an alternate position, you'll miss the perineum rubbing that some of us love so much.

3) To begin, rotate your pelvis forward and backward, rubbing your perineum lightly on the pillow. (The rubbing just feels good and isn't essential to loosen up your lower region.)

4) Be sure to keep your torso and shoulders steady, just rocking your hips forward and backward. To tell if you're rotating instead of just moving, put your hands on your hips pointing down. If the angle of your fingers relative to the floor rotates forward and backward, you've got it.

5) Remember to keep sensing what you're feeling inside. Let subtle pleasurable feelings turn into sound. These exercises can reprogram your nervous system to accept and

rejoice from pleasure if you let them. But they're not supposed to be strenuous calisthenics. It's more like mild Yoga to loosen you up, so your energy channels are freer.

6) After practicing for a few minutes, let the rocking spread up your body like a wave. Imagine you have the body of a snake so that your hip rocking moves upward in an undulating wave.

7) Add in the PC Pump now. Squeeze in one direction of rocking, relax in the other. Due to your brilliant powers of observation, you've probably recognized that there are two ways to do it: pump as you rock forward or pump as you rock back. Which do you like better? Do it the way that you prefer.

Exercise: Orgasmic Breathing

Now you've tried all the separate pieces of Orgasmic Breathing:
- Deep belly breathing through the mouth
- Pelvic rocking
- PC pumping on the inhale
- Making sensual sounds that express pleasure
- Visualizing energy moving up and down your inner flute

I've broken them down into defined steps so you could get comfortable with each one separately. But, once you learn to coordinate them all, Orgasmic Breathing is just doing one unified act. Most people naturally do these things during ecstatic sex, so why not use them consciously? You may have to practice a few times to get the pieces working together. Once you do, just practice this combined exercise every day or two for a few weeks, for 15 minutes at a time.

1) Use whatever position you want.

2) Start breathing.

3) Rock one way on the in-breath, the other on the out-breath.

4) Add the PC pump.

5) Make sounds as you start to feel good.

6) Visualize the energy coming into your first chakra and being pumped up your inner flute by your PC contractions.

7) When you first practice, aim for the heart chakra. Of course, you can practice moving the energy up to any chakra, all the way to the crown of the head. Do what feels best in the moment.

8) Enjoy for a few minutes.

Orgasmic Breathing is the primary method of channeling energy away from vajra when you're making love. It's a major key to Orgasm Mastery techniques that's at the heart of *Male Multiple Orgasm*. Later in this book, there are some partner exercises to develop the knack in the sack.

Exercise: Orgasmic Breathing Self-Pleasuring

Have you noticed yet that many of these exercises are based on earlier skills you developed? Let's combine Orgasmic Breathing with Self-Pleasuring.

Orgasmic Breathing Self-Pleasuring combines giving yourself pleasure with moving the energy from your jewels up your inner flute. Why? Because it should feel good, even better than just doing vajra. Because you get to practice releasing the energy inward and upward instead of outward. Because it's the window to having multiple full-body implosive orgasms without ejaculating. Not a bad sales pitch, don't you think?

1) Create a bit of a ritual with this exercise. Clean your temple (your practice area). Bathe your divine body. Light a candle. Meditate by watching your breath for a few minutes. Set your intention to honor yourself with divine pleasure.

2) Sensuously massage your whole body with loving caresses. Be sure to include your non-genital erogenous zones.

3) Begin Orgasmic Breathing for a few minutes.

4) When you're ready (but not too quickly), begin pleasuring vajra and your entire jewel region. Continue Orgasmic

Breathing while you do this. Take extra special time and care to savor the sweet feelings you're capable of experiencing. Enjoy, don't rush.

5) When you reach an arousal level of 6, focus on moving the sexual energy from your first chakra, up your inner flute, to your heart or higher.

6) Use the techniques that work best for you to channel those orgasmic feelings upward and inward. Slow your rate of breathing. Use your PC to pump energy up on your in-breath. Relax your PC and consciously lower your devamani on your out-breath. Make sounds to release energy. Visualize your sexual energy as a stream of fire getting colder as it goes down your inner flute and out your jewels.

7) Continue pleasuring vajra and your entire body up to arousal level 8, 9, and higher. Use whatever stop-start or interrupting ejaculation tools you choose to keep the fire burning as long as you want without exploding.

A Little Check-In

We're just about done with what you can do yourself. One last main technique, plateauing, remains to help extend your lovemaking stamina. Before we go there, let's do a brief check-in.

If, after repeated practice, you don't feel any energy movement, look back at the earlier exercises and see if you short-circuited something. Maybe one of your fundamental anchors is a little shaky, preventing you from opening to the subtle flows stimulated by Orgasmic Breathing.

If so, look in the Resources section at the back of this book for some tools that can help you increase your sensitivity to subtle energy.

As a result of these exercises, I can honestly say that moving energy is now more pleasurable and desirable to me than a fast suck or hard fuck. And I love sex of all kinds, so that's really saying a lot.

PLATEAUING: THE FINAL SOLO P

The final solo P ability for you to master is plateauing. Remember that the graph of peaking shoots up steeply and then drops quickly? Plateauing will be easy to grasp because it doesn't mean a quick drop.

As the graph on page 39 shows, you move up to a high level of pleasure and then stay there, enjoying it as long as you want. When you can circulate the orgasmic energy up from your lower chakras, you can simply float on a true ecstatic high, basking in the divine light that infuses your whole body.

Once you've experienced a nonstop whole-body orgasm like this, you can understand how the typical male's fascination with wet orgasm pales by comparison. The Male Multiple Orgasm's hidden magic works inside you to replace the urge to ejaculate with something better. If you haven't started to crave more and more from extended self-pleasuring or Orgasmic Breathing, plateauing is a likely place for the shift to begin.

Exercise: Practice Plateauing

I'm not going to be too directive in this exercise because you should have learned what works best for you from all your earlier practice. If needed, use Stop-Start Peaking and other ejaculation interruption techniques as an emergency backup to prevent you from going over the top during this exercise.

But stopping for more than an instant isn't really the idea of plateauing. Here, you want to use your breath, sound, PC pumps, and subtle adjustments to pace yourself and maintain a steady buzz of turn-on. Orgasmic Breathing will become your primary ally for plateauing. Use it to open your inner flute while your arousal level rises, creating an open channel for the energy to stream up and out of your jewels.

By the way, if you skipped some earlier assignments or rushed the parts that didn't appeal to you, congratulations for asserting yourself. But if, after a few tries, you run into a little trouble maintaining a peak for an extended period, you might consider backtracking to the skills you slighted.

1) Self-pleasure vajra up to an arousal level of 6 while doing Orgasmic Breathing (you know, rocking, pumping, moaning, and visualizing).

2) When you reach 6, slow your movements and breathing, using sounds and visualizations to channel the sexual energy up your inner flute.

3) If you keep climbing, slow and deepen your breath even more, and use several PC pumps or other adjustments—like slowing your stroking or moving from vajra's head to shaft.

4) Once you can maintain arousal level 6 for a while, let your arousal rise to an 8 and enjoy leveling at that plateau for a few minutes.

5) Move the energy up your inner flute, swirling it around your heart, or higher to your third eye. Can you feel the energy elsewhere in your body? Focus on it, move around it, and breathe into it to heighten the orgasmic feelings outside your jewels.

6) Now play with maintaining a plateau at 9.

7) You may easily experience a dry orgasm if you plateau high enough and long enough. If your PC starts to spasm all on its own, hold your breath, relax your muscles, and enjoy the ride.

8) Finally, see how long and how close to 9.9 you can ride the wave of pleasure, hovering just before the point of no return.

9) If you slip over the edge, enjoy the gift of orgasmic pleasure, knowing that your search for Orgasm Mastery is nearing its own plateau.

When you find you can maintain a high level of pleasure for an extended period of time, recognize that you've really come a long way, baby. Please be sure to stop and rest some before you continue.

Now You're a Solo Master

Congratulations on completing Solo Mastery. Now you have the tools to engage partners in extended lovemaking.

Honestly, I don't believe you ever graduate from the key practices you've learned here. Relaxation, open senses, PC pumps, pacing, peaking, plateauing, and Orgasmic Breathing are now the essentials of your perpetual personal exercise program. Use it or lose it should be your mantra to stay in shape. Keep it up, all right?

It's again time to report to any intimate partners you play with. Briefly explain what you've practiced, what you felt, and how you expect it will ultimately change your lovemaking.

Of course, next we'll embark on perfecting these skills with a partner. Some of these skills can be and should be maintained through joint practice. Some of them you'll want to come back to now and then when you're without a partner or lose the edge. Others, PC pumps for example, should be part of your daily regimen.

CHAPTER 6

✧ *Partner Prep*

Now you'll begin to integrate your new skills into partner practices. As you gain mastery over the Male Multiple Orgasm, you'll naturally become a much better lover. And you'll enjoy it much more.

Chapter 6 is about more than your needs, since you've got to negotiate a workable deal with a partner, new or long-term. This is not something that works well if you keep it a secret or spring it on a lover while in the sack. So we'll talk about communication before you get to touch each other. Then, you'll take turns pleasuring each other—using your hands at first. You may want to add mouths, lips, and tongues while you're at it. The final exercises in this chapter are about pleasuring each other at the same time. Oh, I almost forgot, without a wet orgasm, at least to start.

I've made a big deal about RAMPER at the beginning of each chapter up to this point. This chapter and Chapter 7 are about how the first five parts, RAMPE, all work together so I'll leave it at that. Use everything you've learned so far and have fun.

ACCEPT YOURSELF
AND THE TRUTH WILL SET YOU FREE

You and I have gotten close through all these intimate exercises, right? I think it's time to be completely honest with ourselves and with each other.

Is it the guy's role to always be up, hard, and long-lasting without exception? Well, some part of me has always wanted that to be so, but the more conscious part of me realizes that it takes two to Tango. We've all got strengths, needs, and limitations. Two basic parts of Male Multiple Orgasm (MMO for short) are capitalizing on your strengths and playing around the weaknesses.

Will you become the world's greatest stud, able to satisfy any and all at any time? Maybe and maybe not. Sometimes, you may find that your biorhythms, energy, or chemistry with a lover just aren't there.

Accept yourself, your strengths and occasional limitations. If you can do that, it will help your lovemaking skills and sexual stamina tremendously.

I'm injecting a strong reality factor here before we begin partner exercises. Want to know why? I'm glad you asked. Because your success will largely depend on the attitude and cooperation of the person you practice with. That means the way you enter into joint exercises with a long-term partner, or how you approach a new one. You both have to be open, aboveboard, and tolerant of mistakes. I've promised to help you talk about this stuff, and I will shortly.

Have a "YES-BE" Attitude

To have reached this point of the MMO program, you've had to love and accept yourself. To go further, you and your partner need to work and play together with a "YES-BE" Attitude.

What is a "YES-BE" Attitude? It's a different way of accepting life, sex, and yourselves, being totally open, totally without resistance.

I use the acronym "YES-BE " to remind us that self-acceptance is purely positive, enhancing our spiritual being. The letters stand for:

Y – Yes, reminding you to allow and accept instead of resisting.

E – **E**xperience now, by watching yourself to raise your consciousness.

S – Love your **S**elf, accepting that your divine nature is good.

B – Be in your **B**ody, not your mind, with open senses, feelings, and heart.

E – **E**njoy pleasure, joy, and sexual energy to remember your basic nature.

When two lovers play with YES-BE, the sky is literally the limit. That's why we're starting this chapter with building a partnership.

PARTNERING GUIDELINES

The best kind of lovemaking is a joint dance where each lover surrenders to inner waves of energy and both assist each other to reach higher and higher peaks. Pleasure, not orgasm, is the aim. By soaring together, each partner can reach unheard-of peaks and plateaus that culminate in bigger, stronger, deeper, often simultaneous spiritual climaxes. But pushing for the Big O puts your attention out of the moment and on the wrong thing.

Of course, yielding to that familiar urge to let loose can short-circuit the whole deal as well.

Common Aims

If your lover is pushing for maximum stimulation and rushing headlong toward orgasm as quickly as possible, the two of you will be playing at cross-purposes. To prevent this, both of you need to agree on common aims based on the MMO vision of lovemaking. This means each of you being totally responsible for your own pleasure, asking for what you want, giving sensitive feedback, going slowly, and savoring physical and intimate delights together. This is how love partners stretch their communion out for long periods of time.

Finding Partners

If you're single and still developing confidence in your Orgasmic Mastery, I understand that you may have some apprehension about entering into a new sexual relationship. The whole communication thing creates its own tensions, which we well know contribute to ejaculating too quickly.

So when you're getting to know someone new and want to have sex, honesty is as important as confidence. Therefore, I strongly urge you to approach this delicate subject candidly before you take your clothes off. This may seem awkward or even daunting, so here are some suggestions to help you approach the conversation frankly, positively, and without putting yourself down.

In other words, I don't want you to blurt out "I come too quickly" in a spurt of honesty. Remember, that's the old you, one we don't want to reinforce.

Here are some sample opening lines to broach this subject. Feel free to modify them so it sounds like you talking. Just be sure to make it positive...

"I'm studying to be a Tantric lover, merging spirit with physical pleasure. Tantra is an ancient spiritual practice that uses sexual energy to raise consciousness. It's teaching me to view sex as a sacred meditation.

"What this all means is that I want to go slowly, learning how to worship your body as I'm learning to love and appreciate your soul. You excite me tremendously, but I don't want to get swept away too soon, rushing toward a quick release. I'd rather begin by playing sensitively with the energy between us for long periods of time and move forward without any goals other than pleasure.

"Will you dance with me, letting us experiment and teach each other, communicating each step of the way so we can know each other fully and intimately?"

If you have success with your own version of this dialogue, or run into problems, please email me at somraj@tantraattahoe.com and let me know.

Long-Term Partners

Clearly, men with long-term partners have someone close at hand to practice with. This obvious advantage may be accompanied by some drawbacks. If involuntary ejaculation has been a problem for some time, as wonderful as your partner may be, some emotional issues might surface when you broach the subject of MMO Sex and Orgasm Mastery.

The emotions you might be met with—hesitance, resentment, disbelief, apathy, infuriation—can seem illogical until you develop some empathy for your lover's situation. If you overreact to these emotions, you could blow the whole deal before you get started. Here are some suggestions that may help you to look at things from their viewpoint:

- Consider the way your long-term lover might be compensating for the state of your love life. Your partner might value other emotional needs—security, affection, companionship—more than complete physical satisfaction. People have been known to live happily ever after while giving up something elusive (big orgasms) in exchange for something that's important to them (like having those emotional needs met). If you propose changing this dynamic, in one sense you're refusing to accept that sacrifice. If you think this might be the case, discuss how you value what your partner has done in the past and how these emotional needs could be met along with better sex.
- Maybe sexual union isn't your partner's favorite activity. Maybe you're the one who's way more interested in sex. If either is the case, it makes sense that your MMO program may not seem worth your partner's effort. I wonder if your partner has ever really experienced ecstatic sex? If not, see

if you can get your lover's interest in the prospect of something much, much better.

- Your partner may have concerns and objections to some of the consequences of the Male Multiple Orgasm program. For example, extended lovemaking can cause soreness. Of course, the slow stop-start beginning is a good way to counter this concern. If sensitive tissues are an issue, you need to promise to be extra careful, conscious, and assertive about replenishing lubrication.

- A structured approach doesn't work for everybody. Your partner may worry that you'll become too clinical in bed and lose whatever heart-centered spontaneity you have. If so, explain that the structure is a temporary phase designed to permanently enhance your spontaneous lovesharing. You can also propose to alternate making love with and without structure while going through this program.

- Some partners might react with a "What's in it for me?" Explain the promise of extended spiritual bliss. Or horse-trade if you have to, offering to do something your partner finds valuable. In other words, make a deal that works for both of you.

- Your partner's fears may get in the way. Fear of failure or fear of being blamed for failure can block your chances of winning cooperation. Here's where relating the great strides you've made can help. That's why I've been urging regular check-ins throughout the Male Multiple Orgasm program. Reassure your lover of the 95% chance of success and that you won't hold anything against them.

- Feeling coerced into helping or pressured into participating is no way to build a willing intimate partnership. If your lover feels this way, you need to go out of your way to let them make the choice entirely. Taking personal responsibility and always enlisting the other's permission are fundamental principles of MMO.

- It's not uncommon for people to resist change. Resistance like this often causes hidden insecurities to surface. Your partner might think: "If he can last forever, will he still need me?" Reassure your partner that you're doing this program partly to strengthen your love relationship, adding a powerful bonding energy you haven't experienced very often. Sometimes just broaching the subject lightly and letting it sit for a while is enough to overcome resistance to change.

- Your partner may worry that your desire for better love-making skills is a ticket to swinging or polyamory (a lifestyle with open multiple lovers). Explain that the majority of couples are blissfully monogamous and that's the right style for you. (If they read parts of this book, you might want to downplay my own polyamorous lifestyle, which isn't a goal of this program.)

If other fears or objections come up, please email me at somraj@tantraattahoe.com and let me know.

What overall approach do you need to take to negotiate a cooperative partnership for the Male Multiple Orgasm?

- Above all, enter into the discussion with patience MMO mindset of total gratitude for the gifts of the Goddess.

- Let your partner choose to play or not—never use force, pressure, or manipulation to enlist your lover's help.

- Continue to provide reassurance of your love and commitment to the relationship.

- Make it clear that this program is designed to be a joint experience of deeper intimacy and bonding, giving you both everything you ever dreamed of.

- Finally, believe and explain to your partner that once you've both experienced higher and higher waves of ecstasy together through MMO lovemaking, any memory of these concerns will pass away quickly.

If, for any reason, broaching these topics is too touchy for you, seriously consider some sessions with a qualified local sex therapist.

Your Role

Your role in partner play begins with being able to receive pleasure. At first glance, that may SOUND easy. I'm talking about relaxing, emptying your mind of doubt, rising above your fears, letting yourself go, and forgetting about reciprocating for the moment. We all seem to have programmed limits of how much pleasure we're willing to experience and how receptive we're able to be. Giving pleasure is a big turn-on to me so I've had to learn how to simply relax while allowing my partner to just give me pleasure. All of this is easier said than done, don't you agree?

Your first assignment here is to establish the intention to surrender to receiving pleasure. Be conscious of your limits and reactions. When you run into an internal barrier, be willing to stop and talk about it calmly. The sooner you do this, the less emotional it usually is.

Next, you've got to be an open book. You've been checking in with your partner regularly, reporting your progress, and sharing the downs as well as the ups, right? If not, it's time to start communicating lots more about this program. We've talked about the big downside of hiding your MMO practices from your partner. Secrecy breeds tension, which breeds involuntary ejaculation. Not only will your behavior seem strange to a lover who doesn't understand where you're coming from, but they may get too wild and push for orgasm while you're developing the knack of lasting.

Last, you need to trust your partner on occasion to take complete charge. Trust builds gradually and organically so this is not an easy feeling to mandate. If you've been talking about this program and your partner has been listening supportively, you've made a good start. Read each exercise together carefully before you begin. Regardless, the first exercises in this chapter wade into sensual sharing cautiously. As you begin together, keep your expectations low and take it slow. Repeat each practice enough times until you both begin to feel confident with each other's commitment to make the program work. Setbacks are expected, and when they occur, the best thing to do is to backtrack to the last exercise you did successfully together.

Partner's Role

Lovers with a deep heart-to-heart connection will inherently want the best for each other. With agreement on the vision of MMO Lovemaking, they'll naturally accept the roles being spelled out here. But lovers who believe that they're totally at fault for their partner's jewel sensitivity and hair trigger may be reluctant to fully engage. Both must own their share of the situation openly.

A partner who feels completely responsible for their lovers' pleasure might push for explosive orgasms to prove their love. The desire to make a guy climax works as strongly on some women as it does on us guys. Lovers insecure about their sexuality may feel that making their partner let loose proves that they're sexy, desirable, and skilled in bed. If you find yourself in this situation, explain about voluntary ejaculation, implosive energy orgasms, and that ultimately we're each the master of our own ecstasy.

Lovers who don't have orgasms easily may, when they get close, lose themselves in a rush toward explosive relief, dragging their partners over the edge. They need to understand about the advantages of playing without goals, and how bigger and better orgasms may eventually result. Explain how basking in the flood of excitement in each moment lets the energy build to higher and higher plateaus.

Without this frank kind of dialogue, your partner may push you into a style of sex that won't work for you early in the program, or ever. To prevent this from happening, tell your lover how much more pleasure you'll both receive by starting slowly. Mention the pleasure you receive from IMPLOSIVE orgasms. Remind your beloved that you'll be less sensitive after one of these inner energy experiences and ready to stroke faster and deeper for a while. Above all else, let your partner know that you can go to unheard-of altered states together through MMO love-making by changing the rules of the game of sex.

To Let Loose or Not

We sensitive guys may still have the familiar urge to ejaculate as our occasional or constant companion. Even if you've begun to experience something better than a quick release, old programming sometimes dies hard. So, before we begin partner exercises, we'd be well-advised to address the age-old question: "To let loose or not?" With a partner in the mix, answering becomes a more complex dynamic.

You realize that I'm pro-ejaculation, in general, because I strongly believe that pleasure in all forms is a good thing. So maybe you'll accept my suggestion of moderation in good grace. I think it's a good idea for the two of you to commit that neither will intentionally go for the Big O during practice sessions without open agreement first. Be sure to discuss the consequences of the Male Multiple Orgasm's learning strategy: how getting close to the point of no return repeatedly will cause mistakes. You need to learn to read each other's signals and collaborate together to stay in the bliss plateau. Also, it would be great to make a deal that you'll both enjoy all orgasms together, whether dry or wet, intentional or accidental, and sometimes go for it.

TURNING EACH OTHER ON

MMO Lovemaking is complex because it requires managing your own stimulation while responding to your partner's signals. Your mind can be full of questions like:

"Is what I'm doing working?"

"What do I do next?"

"Am I getting too close?"

"Is my partner getting close?"

That's why we begin Male Multiple Orgasm partner training by alternating giving and receiving. When you're receiving, you can completely focus your full attention on your outer sensations, your inner feelings, and your own pleasure. To make progress, you'll have to fully accept being in this receptive role.

Achieving this is a learning experience all by itself for most guys who are programmed to be the ultimate satisfier of women.

Satisfying Each Other—One at a Time

You'd be wise to expect some adjustment as you settle into pure receptivity. If you can remember some hot experiences when your lover simply gave to you, it will be easier to make an agreement about satisfying each other one at a time. When you each know full well that you'll return the favor later, it will be easier to relax and surrender.

Before doing each practice, be sure you read the instructions together. Except for the first couple of exercises in this chapter, which are clearly marked, you'll want to do most of these practices several times, spread over a week or two. Remember, you're absorbing the MMO spirit of lovemaking, which advises you to go slowly and savor every little tidbit of sensation. Focus on the journey, not the destination. Don't rush, so you can enjoy more.

Exercise: Agreeing on Signals

Take a few minutes now to agree on signals you'll depend on during practices and unstructured lovemaking. Signals are words, sounds, or hand motions you'll use to give your partner feedback about your erotic reactions and arousal level. You'll both benefit from having a crystal-clear shorthand that lets you express yourself without getting too deeply into the mind. It takes practice to ensure a quick, simple, effortless, non-distracting way to alert your partner to where you're at in each moment.

Primary among these cues is your version of the 10-point scale we've been using (see page 36):

1) Read the instructions to this exercise together.

2) Agree on words, sounds, or signals for "slow" and "stop." I like to say "slower" or "I'm close" to slow my partner down, and sometimes I put my hands up in a stopping motion. Some lovers like to squeeze their partner's hips or shoulders lightly, push upward, or grab their hands to ask for a complete stop. Feel free to invent your own and use what feels best.

3) Explain your experience with the 10-point scale and any personal definitions you've discovered. Agree that sometimes you'll just use a number to convey your level of arousal.

4) Practice with a communication cycle that begins and ends with positive reinforcement. I call this the "feedback sandwich." It's a diplomatic way to ask for changes without hurting your partner's feelings. Anytime you want to be pleasured differently, begin by finding something to compliment. Next, ask for what you want, explaining how that would feel even better. Finally, acknowledge something about what's working. For example, if your partner is stroking vajra too lightly, you might say...

"You have the most delicate hands."

"This would feel even better with more pressure."

"Ooooh, that's really exciting. Thanks."

If the change isn't exactly what you were asking for, do another three-step feedback sandwich. Practice the feedback cycle now by exchanging back scratching until you feel comfortable using the three steps routinely.

5) Practice "yes/no" questions. During erotic play, we all sink into speechless times when the feedback sandwich

would be difficult to do. While deep in the throes of ecstasy, too much explaining and verbalizing can spoil the mood. Asking open-ended questions (such as "How does this feel?") may shift your lover's attention out of their body and into formulating an appropriate response. When my partner isn't giving me any feedback, I've learned to ask one-word questions that can be answered with a simple "yes" or "no" or shake of the head. I use yes/no questions to better understand how I'm doing and what I could do better. Use simple questions like...

"Faster?" "Slower?" "Harder?" "Softer?"

Practice yes/no questions now by exchanging neck or head rubs.

6) Talk frankly about the fact that, because you want to push the envelope, sometimes you'll go over 9.9 and ejaculate. Agree on any signals that work for you to alert your partner how close you are and when you've gone too far. Be sure you acknowledge that the Male Multiple Orgasm is all about pleasure. Find a way to accept that a wet release is part of the fun.

7) Briefly discuss with your partner any other situations that come to mind that you feel you need signals for.

When you first do this exercise, don't try to plan for every possible circumstance. Go through Agreeing On Signals at an introductory level first. Come back to it later if you need more clarity and better signals for new situations.

Exercise: How I Like to Be Loved

The more you practice and play together, the more you learn about what turns each other on. Even long-time lovers don't know everything that's going on inside their partners at each moment.

You've learned a tremendous amount about your erogenous zones and arousal patterns from the previous solo exercises. For the fastest results with Male Multiple Orgasm, you need to share as much of this with your practice partner as you can—quickly and comfortably. As well, turnabout is fair play. The more you each educate your beloved about what works for you and what doesn't, the better you'll both be able to read each other.

That's what the "How I Like to Be Loved" exercise is all about: teaching your partner your erogenous zones and what turns you on the most. It's like the Whole Body Sensory Focus exercise with your beloved watching. Some people find touching themselves in front of another even more challenging than other forms of lovemaking. But to practice extending orgasm together, you need to grow into this deeper level of intimacy. Does it help you to approach this as a demonstration of the Orgasm Mastery that you've developed from the previous exercise program?

If you find this to be too awkward, don't push it too fast. Talk about your feelings openly before you begin. Go slowly, do a little at a time, take breaks, breathe deeply, and relax all you can. This whole program will gradually elevate your intimacy to a new level. Now is the best time to start.

1) Create a comfortable sacred space to relax naked in front of your partner.

2) Touch your body lightly, slowly, and gently, avoiding your jewels at first, like you did during the Whole Body Sensory Focus exercise in Chapter 4. Demonstrate what you like and don't like all over your body, explaining any feelings and sensations as they occur.

3) Next, self-pleasure vajra showing what you like and what you've learned from the Self-Pleasuring Discovery exercise in Chapter 4. Especially demonstrate the strokes you prefer and the ones you don't like as much.

4) Help your partner understand that watching you closely is top priority. Comment on what you're doing as you do it, where your attention is at each moment, how different movements feel, and what's changing inside such as PC

pumps and inner vibrations. Make sure your partner notices changes in your breathing, sounds, hardness, color, testicle elevation, spasms, and other symptoms of running energy.

5) Be sure to continually comment on your arousal level using the 10-point scale.

6) Then ask your partner to do the same exercise, demonstrating preferred techniques and maximum turn-ons. Fair is fair, right?

7) If you want to take this exercise all the way to a wet release, agree on a second phase of the joint exercise similar to the Ejaculation Awareness you practiced solo in Chapter 4. While you get yourself off, describe everything that's going on, inside and out, to the best of your ability in the moment or as soon afterward as possible.

8) Alternately, you can do the exercise at the same time, turning it into a mutual self-pleasuring experience. Aim to bring yourselves up to three peaks together without climaxing. If you want to go all the way, practice timing your orgasms to see what it takes to make them happen together.

I find this last step much more exciting than private self-pleasuring. If it's the same for you, you may find that it makes you even more sensitive than normal. So you may slip and have to practice more. That's a good thing, right? Some couples find great excitement in repeating step 8 frequently as just another way to honor pleasure.

If you are comfortable and thorough, you probably only need to do the first parts of the "How I Like To Be Loved" exercise once right now. It's a great thing to repeat between stages of the program after you've learned more about yourself and your sensuality. Besides, over time we change. After years of Tantric LovePlay, Jeffre and I still learn new things this way about what turns each other on.

Exercise: Partner Whole Body Sensory Focus

Early in the Male Multiple Orgasm process, you practiced becoming more aware of your body and senses. In this exercise, you'll exchange gentle exploratory massage like you did in your solo Whole Body Sensory Focus. This is just another step in learning to shift your focus to other erogenous zones so all your energy doesn't just reside in your jewels. Also, it's great training to be more active with your whole body during sex. By using full-body caresses and non-jewel touching, you can learn to avoid fixating on just the hardest and wettest spots alone.

1) Lie down nude in a relaxed posture in a safe, comfortable, uninterrupted space, with your partner sitting comfortably by your side. If you own a massage table, you may prefer to use it for this exercise.

2) Take a few deep belly breaths to relax and let go of any stress you've been carrying.

3) Ask your partner to be the giver first. Ask your sweetie to LIGHTLY and slowly touch your whole body, excluding your jewels. Your partner will want to use what some call a "taking touch." This means that the giver feels as much with the touching hand as the receiver does with the part that's being caressed. By taking touch, the giver concentrates on energy flowing to and from the heart, through the arms, into the hands and fingers. Doc Steven says about this: "If you're touching the skin, you're too close. If you're not touching, you're too far." You, as receiver, can guide your partner's touch by making sounds on the out-breath to let the giver know where to concentrate.

4) Have your giver explore your body gently and SLOWLY, except for your jewels, as if a young child with a new toy. Let your partner experiment with different strokes on different body parts, feeling each sensation as though for the first time. The giver can use fingertips, finger backs, nails, palms, backs of hands, forearms, and even hair. Ask your

giver to mix different speeds and different pressures with different body parts. The giver can touch like a spider walking slowly on the skin, like a butterfly wandering aimlessly, and like a moth dancing around a flame. This is a good place for your giver to practice asking yes/no questions to get guidance on what's occurring.

5) Ask your partner to pay special attention to massaging your face, hands, and feet, one at a time, of course. Releasing tension from these areas, while not always sexually arousing, can be tremendously relaxing. For example, some experts report that letting go of the mask of facial tension we all carry goes a long way toward helping us overcome the internal stress that contributes to involuntary release.

6) Use the feedback sandwich to ask for changes. Even if everything is perfect, practice asking for changes a couple of times.

7) Next, have your partner do a similar exploration with your jewels. Yes, I mean your vajra and devamani (your penis and testicles), and anywhere around there that turns you on. Together, explore your favorite parts lightly and slowly in the same childlike way without trying to ejaculate. If this turns you on and you get hard, well, that's great! Show it proudly.

8) Then, ask your partner to include your whole body in the same way, excluding nothing. Feel those excited feelings fully and let your partner know about them through sound and movement. Explain how being turned-on affects different parts of your body: hair, nipples, devamani, vajra, etc.

9) Exchange roles and do the same exercise for your partner.

Do some version of this almost every time you make love. This is an important exercise to do repeatedly. When you can fully relax and feel everything, then it's time to move on.

TAKING TURNS

Together, you and your partner can learn a lot about extending loveplay by exchanging the kind of erotic touching taught in the following exercises. It's also great fun and a way to improve your communication skills—while providing some awesome pleasure.

Exercise: Stop-Start Hand Job

You've got lots of experience with the solo version of the Stop-Start Hand Job Exercise. Remember Stop-Start Peaking from your work self-pleasuring (is that an oxymoron?) in Chapters 4 and 5. You have the same aim here: enjoying 30 minutes of stroking without a wet release. All you have to do now is bring your partner into the swing of things, let them take over the arduous task of massaging vajra, and get coordinated.

1) Lie on your back in your most comfortable position: have your knees bent, supported by a pillow, or simply extended straight out. Your partner can sit or kneel between your legs or at your side. Giver comfort is as important as receiver comfort. Tension in the giver's body transmits to the receiver, so be sure to experiment and find a position that can last awhile for both of you.

2) After preliminaries like talking, relaxing, breathing, and full-body sensual massage, ask your partner to begin stroking vajra and your devamani with unlubricated hands.

3) Your partner should closely watch for signs of your rising arousal: vajra's hardness and color, breathing changes, thrusting hips, body jerks, lifting of devamani, pulsing of vajra or pelvic muscles, hands pushing away, and withdrawing pelvis. At the same time as your partner observes you closely, you should be giving verbal feedback about your sensations and level of arousal.

4) When you reach arousal level 6 on the scale, use whatever signal you've agreed on so that your partner immediately stops all stimulation. You may want to ask your

lover's hands be removed entirely if that helps you relax. You know the rest of the drill: open your eyes wide, relax all your muscles, take slow deep breaths, and wait until your excitement drops to arousal level 2.

5) Repeat steps (2) through (4) five more times up to arousal level 6.

6) Continue the exercise by repeating the same steps up to an arousal level 8. Then do it all again up to arousal level 9.

7) When you can receive a hand job for 30 minutes by stopping and starting without ejaculating, repeat steps 2 through 7 with your honey's hands being lubricated.

8) If you want to push it, agree with your partner that you want to see how close you can come to 9.9, knowing full well that you're likely to slip over the edge and explode. Enjoy it and, like I said before, literally squeeze every last drop of pleasure out of vajra.

9) Exchange roles and manually pleasure your partner, following the guidance you receive. If your partner is a woman, follow her instructions carefully, since I haven't included any female anatomy or stroking techniques in this volume.

When you can enjoy high peaks while your partner is pleasuring vajra with lubrication for 30 minutes or more, move on to the next exercise.

Exercise: Subtle Adjustments Hand Job

Now that you have some confidence about backing off with your partner's help, it's time to move on to Subtle Adjustments Peaking. Here, you'll repeat the previous exercise except you'll ask your partner to make small changes in how vajra is being pleasured instead of stopping entirely. Your communication skills will become even more essential now. Take full advantage of your signals, feedback sandwich, and yes/no questions.

1) Use a comfortable position for both of you.

2) After preliminaries like talking, relaxing, breathing, and full-body sensual massage, ask your partner to begin stroking vajra and your devamani with unlubricated hands.

3) Ask your partner to experiment with different strokes, speeds, and pressures to find what's more and less pleasurable just as you did during Self-Pleasuring Discovery. Have your partner:

- Alternate hands to see which feels better.
- Try upward strokes, downward strokes, thumb forward and thumb back.
- Concentrate on the shaft, on the head (glans or crown), and the frenulum (the sensitive underside of the head).
- Use thumb and forefinger as a ring upward and downward, with thumb forward and back.
- Roll vajra between both hands like a rolling pin, and use both hands from mid-shaft out or from top and bottom to middle.
- Rub vajra's underside with the flat of the hand, and press or roll vajra against your belly or thigh.
- Pull or tickle your devamani with the other hand.
- Use the corkscrew, rotating the hand as it slides up, and the pop-off, squeezing while suddenly pulling the hand up and over vajra's head.

Some of these may be rough or uncomfortable without lubrication. If you find that to be the case, do the comfortable ones first and then use oil or cream for the remaining ones.

4) When you reach arousal level 6, instead of stopping stimulation, ask your partner to vary the strokes to reduce your excitement level a few points (for example, from arousal level 6 down to a 4). Suggest that your partner slow down, lighten the pressure, change direction, move

from the head to the shaft, shorten the strokes, or use other moves that are less exciting.

5) Follow the same regimen as Stop-Start Peaking, repeating each series six times up to arousal level 6, 8, and 9, or higher.

6) When you can enjoy vajra being pleasured for 30 minutes using subtle adjustments to drop your excitement level a few points, ask your partner to repeat the whole process with lubricated hands.

7) If you want to push it, agree with your partner that you want to see how close you can come to arousal level 9.9, knowing full well that you're likely to slip over the edge and explode.

8) Exchange roles and manually pleasure your partner, carefully following the guidance you receive.

When you can enjoy high peaks without stopping or ejaculating while your partner is pleasuring vajra with lubrication for 30 minutes or more, move on to the next exercise. Now you're very close to reality, since we'll be using Subtle Adjustments Peaking during sexual union later in the Male Multiple Orgasm program.

Exercise: Breath Peaking Hand Job

So much in this chapter is already familiar to you. Now you're going to use Orgasmic Breathing to spread your excitement away from your hot spots like you did in the solo Breath Peaking exercise.

1) Use a comfortable position for both of you.

2) After preliminaries like talking, relaxing, breathing, and full-body sensual massage, ask your partner to begin stroking vajra and your devamani slowly. You decide whether you want to start with dry or lubricated hands, depending on how sensitive you feel and how well you've been doing with previous mastery exercises.

3) When you reach arousal level 6, instead of stopping stimulation, ask your partner to slow down slightly. Open your eyes wide, inhale more deeply into the belly, but this time through the NOSE, and hold your breath.

4) Relax completely as you exhale, visualizing your sexual fire streaming out of vajra, and moaning with pleasure to release energy.

5) Inhale again through the nose, visualizing that pleasurable energy moving up vajra through your pelvis to your heart and higher. Use one long or several short PC Pumps to help you shoot the energy upward.

6) Can you feel your excitement lessen simply by slowing your breath? Play with it until you can. See how long you can maintain a high plateau while you adjust your breathing. Use techniques to interrupt ejaculation if you need to. Guide your partner to use stop-start and subtle adjustments as required.

7) Follow the same regimen as with the peaking exercises, repeating each series six times up to arousal level 6, 8, and 9, or higher.

8) As you practice and get closer and closer to ejaculation, see if you can back off your arousal level just by slowing and deepening your breath without your partner changing anything. When you can balance on the very edge of 9.9, you're bound to experience implosive orgasms, where you vibrate inside and stream the energy upward without a wet release.

9) Exchange roles and manually pleasure your partner, carefully following the guidance you receive.

Exercise: Oral Pleasuring

Here is an optional exercise, which follows the same sequence of steps as above but using oral pleasuring. I call it optional because not everyone loves oral sex. If you're willing, it's another great way to develop Orgasm Mastery in a highly exciting situation.

1) Use a comfortable position for both of you.

2) After preliminaries like talking, relaxing, breathing and full-body sensual massage, ask your partner to slowly begin licking and sucking your vajra and devamani.

3) When you reach arousal level 6, use whatever signal you've agreed on so that your partner immediately stops all stimulation. You may want to ask for your lover's mouth to be removed entirely if that helps you relax. You know the rest of the drill: open your eyes wide, relax all your muscles, take slow deep breaths, and wait until your excitement drops.

4) Repeat the exercise using Stop-Start at arousal level 6, 8, and 9, six times at each arousal level.

5) Repeat the exercise up to arousal level 6, 8, and 9, guiding your partner with feedback to use Subtle Adjustments to help you peak and then plateau.

6) Repeat the exercise up to arousal level 6, 8, and 9, using Orgasmic Breathing to help you peak and then plateau.

7) As you practice and get closer and closer to ejaculation, see if you can back off your arousal level just by slowing and deepening your breath without your partner changing anything. When you can balance on the very edge of 9.9, you're bound to experience implosive orgasms, where you vibrate inside and stream the energy upward without a wet release.

8) Exchange roles and orally pleasure your partner, carefully following the guidance you receive.

PLEASURING EACH OTHER
AT THE SAME TIME

We're really upping the ante when you give and receive at the same time. If you're anything like most of the sexy guys I know, giving pleasure turns you on almost as much as receiving.

Pleasuring each other together is a double whammy for really sensitive guys like us. But you've made it this far and have all the requisite skills, right? So let's go for it and play together. What do you say?

Exercise: Mutual Hand Jobs

You've learned an awful lot about your own and your partner's turn-ons. Surely, that's given you greater awareness and confidence in and around sex. For this exercise, though, forget about being too clinical with all that information you've filed away in your mind. Instead, just play in the moment. Act like little kids exploring new territory for the first time.

1) Find a comfortable position where you can lie down next to each other, talk easily, and reach each other's jewels with your hands.

2) Talk about what you've both discovered that you enjoy as if you've just discovered it.

3) Gently caress each other's body, taking pleasure from your touch all over. As you feel it, begin Orgasmic Breathing, including sounds and PC pumps.

4) Slowly begin to focus on each other's jewels, asking yes/no questions and using the feedback sandwich to guide each other.

5) Decide what arousal levels you want to peak at. Give feedback about your arousal level, asking or signaling for stops when you want to peak several times.

6) Continue peaking several times using subtle adjustments and Orgasmic Breathing alone, seeing how long you can make it last.

7) If you want to climax together, go for it and enjoy it.

Repeat this exercise several times until you can use everything you've learned while pleasuring each other.

Exercise: 69

Again, here's another exercise optional for those who delight in oral gratification. If you're willing, 69 may be the most challenging assignment for your MMO Lovemaking partnership, since oral sex limits the amount of talking you can do. You'll be depending more on your ability to channel energy and your partner's ability to read your arousal level.

1) Find a comfortable position where you can each orally pleasure your partner's jewels.

2) Gently caress and sensually massage each other's bodies to get turned on.

3) Slowly begin to focus on each other's jewels.

4) Give lots of nonverbal feedback using moans and movements.

5) If you get too close, pull out. Stop and talk about how you can peak and plateau more easily before continuing.

6) See how long you can make it last by going slowly and using everything you've learned so far.

7) If you want to orgasm together, go for it and enjoy it.

Repeat this exercise several times until you feel adept at using all your Orgasm Mastery tools while pleasuring each other.

Congratulations, my friend! If you've done the exercises to this point, you are totally prepared for the ultimate experience with the Male Multiple Orgasm. I hope you've enjoyed the trip so far. It only gets better once you get inside, as I'm sure you know.

CHAPTER 7

✧ *Longer-Lasting Lovemaking*

Do you agree that sexual union is more stimulating than other kinds of sexual play? Most do, which is why after all your practice, you've now moved up to grad school. If you find manual or oral stimulation more exciting, then what's coming should be easier than the previous chapter.

THE REAL THING?

Some would say that Chapter 7 is about "fucking." Some would say it's about the real thing. In Male Multiple Orgasm, nothing is really profane, but we do prefer to call fucking sexual union. You see, to us, anything that creates the rapturous dance of ecstatic peaks and spiritual plateaus is what we call the real thing. We'll get to some of that during your graduation in the next chapter.

But you have arrived at the chapter that is all about lasting during sexual penetration. That's pretty darn real if you ask me. I call the exercises that follow "VIY" for **V**ajra-**I**n-**Y**oni. Of course, we accept anything that gets your orgasmic energy running— whether it's fucking, sucking, touching, or meditating—as Spiritual Sex.

After a little talk about taking it slowly and choosing the best initial sexual position, we'll begin with several exercises where vajra gets to approach yoni gradually. Then we'll do some very familiar exercises: Stop-Start, Subtle Adjustments, and Orgasmic Breathing. You see how all your intensive practice to date will now pay off in the sack? Before we experiment with all sorts of sexual positions, I'm also going to include some Taoist techniques in which you vary your strokes to prolong lovemaking. Oooh, what fun!

The Smart Sex Talk

It's vital that you consider and discuss smart sex with a new partner before doing these exercises. Even if your partner is a woman who uses birth control pills or another device, YOU need to be responsible to avoid the possible spread of STDs (sexually transmitted diseases). See Chapter 9 for some detailed information about making sex as safe as possible.

No matter your situation and skill level, you'll want to take precautions against unwanted pregnancies. If you're with a long-time monogamous partner and you're sure that you've both been completely faithful, you probably feel secure making love without condoms for STD protection. If you're with a newer partner, I recommend two sets of tests for STDs, including a test for HIV (the AIDS virus), at least three months apart, before playing freely. Regardless of your situation, I strongly recommend that you talk candidly and honestly about pregnancy and STD protection. Then, make a clear, mutually comfortable, agreement before you begin.

Patience, My Friend

Although the Male Multiple Orgasm methods are extremely effective, it might require weeks of practice before you get it just right. Some say this is a six-month program.

Oh, no, not weeks or months of making love over and over again?

Yes, I'm afraid so. Again, it's doctor's orders. Most sex therapists agree that if you're willing to bite the bullet and practice enough, your chances are 95% in favor of developing the confidence to last longer.

However long it takes, hurrying can only build tension and slow you down. Compared to how long you've been slipping past 9.9 without choice and how many decades of extended sexual play you have ahead of you, what's a few months of playing with fire?

You get my point? You've heard it before. Be patient and don't put too much pressure on yourself. That's an order! Got it?

If you don't succeed beyond your wildest dreams the first few times, please shrug it off and remember that you're working toward something that's not a quick fix. It's a "baby steps" kind of deal. Yeah, I've gotten pretty good at what's in this book. And if you knew about how far down some of the downs were, you'd probably feel better about messing up now and then. This is a tortoise and the hare kind of game, you realize? It's a commitment to persistence that pays off, and the goal is not rapid perfection.

If you still have trouble after weeks of practice, don't hesitate to contact a sex therapist for some extra guidance in order to close the deal.

To Foreplay or Not to Foreplay?

You might be tempted to do these VIY (Vajra-In-Yoni) exercises without foreplay. I used to believe that the less stimulation I received before inserting vajra the better, hoping the initial abstinence would make me last longer. I was wrong. Maybe I lasted a few extra minutes, but I would soon rise to a peak very quickly and climax anyway. That was before I knew how to run energy and enjoy myself in a variety of ways for extended periods of time.

Now, I really desire lots of whole-body foreplay to get my energy moving first, like the typical woman. When I start by getting revved up into that pleasure zone where I just want to float with ecstatic feelings swirling throughout my body forever, slow-at-first penetration is fantastic for both of us. If we only have time or energy for a quickie and we rush penetration, I often find that it's just a biological experience. We call that a "first-chakra" event.

Don't get me wrong, I like all kinds of sex. But now I realize that it's risky to us highly sensitive types to begin sexual play while our energy is concentrated in our jewels. Besides, since quick jewel play doesn't turn me on all over, whole-body implosive orgasms are unlikely. I guess you can see why I'm such an ardent fan of foreplay. Of course, as with any suggestions in this book, feel free to try your own approach and do what works best for you.

How Often Do You Do It?

While we're on the subject of foreplay, let's take a moment to consider the effect of frequency of lovemaking on sexual stamina. You know what I mean—how often you do it affects how long you can do it.

If you make love every day or two, not only do your skills stay sharp, but you loosen up and spread the energy that naturally concentrates in your first chakra. If you only make love every week or two, you'll be collecting and storing your sexual juices down there. If you've been without a lover for months, then that first time together will probably be way explosive.

When you're sitting on a reservoir of orgasmic electricity, you're certainly more sensitive and likely to explode easily.

This isn't supposed to be a sales pitch for moving in together. It's just another liberal dose of reality. If your sex life is sporadic, the baggage you'll carry to your encounters will be full of explosive charges.

What should you do about it? The obvious response is practice with a partner more often if you've got one. If you don't have time, then you might want to examine your priorities. If sacred sex is taking a backseat to other energies in your life, then mastery of the moment will be harder to achieve. In this case, you might say you're getting what you planned for.

Frequent self-pleasuring to stimulate and run energy can help. I'm primarily talking about the kind of play that culminates in implosive orgasms. Of course, using ejaculation to blow off the energy that accumulates can make you less excitable when you finally do connect with a partner. But somehow, getting yourself off probably won't calm an excitable system. You'll likely need to regularly merge with female energy to stay in the flow.

Regardless of how hard we try, we all sometimes end up separated from our partners for days or weeks. In this situation, my advice is to take it easy and cut yourself some slack. Let your partner know how excitable you are and expect you'll need to go real slowly. Sometimes you and your partner may just agree on a blow-out explosive orgasm to clean out your chakras. Then, some time later, you can more comfortably relax into the sacred space of ecstatic love play.

SEXUAL POSITIONS

The position you're in during sexual union (intercourse) can affect how long you can go without ejaculating. Let's take a look at your options and consider the effect they have on your stimulation and staying power.

The Seven Basic *Kama Sutra* Sexual Positions

Here are the seven basic sexual positions adapted from the *Kama Sutra*:

- **Shakti** Position (woman on top)
- **Shiva** Position (man on top)
- **Kneeling** Position (man between woman's legs)
- **Transverse** Position (side-to-side)
- **Cow** Position (rear entry)
- **Yab-Yum** Position (sitting)
- **Dancing** Position (standing)

And then there's the comfort and relaxation quotient of each position. Yab-Yum and Dancing Positions are challenging to hold for any length of time. The more effort it takes to maintain a position, the less comfortable you'll be—which can influence how long you can last.

Maybe even more important is what strokes are used. The depth, speed, and angle of yoni penetration will affect vajra's sensitivity. Exactly what parts of vajra get the most friction is critical. And then there's the decision about who's in control of the stroking. When I'm close I like to be in the Transverse, Shiva, or Kneeling Positions so I can choose how fast and how deep to stroke.

There are many variations on these basic stances that influence tightness and freedom to move. So you see, a simple list like this taken from the *Kama Sutra* doesn't tell each individual the positions where *he'll* last the longest. Experimenting is the order of the day, which defines what the exercises in this chapter are all about.

Bummer, you've got to try out a bunch of sexual positions and see what works best for you both.

Who's on First & Who's on Top

The name for the *Kama Sutra* position with the man on top is derived from one of the primary Hindu male gods, "Shiva." Most experts teach that this typical "missionary" position with the man on top of his partner is not the best to extend lovemaking.

When you're on top, you have to support your weight. This generates muscle tension in your arms, shoulders, back, and legs. Along with the added excitement, thrusting motions increase this tension and cause more fatigue. Like most guys, you'll probably clench your pelvis, butt, stomach, and rosetta while pumping from above. All of this can reduce relaxation and increase your chance of slipping past 9.9 against your will.

We call the woman-on-top position "Shakti" after the Tantric name for the Goddess. Experts say that many men find it easier to prolong lovemaking with the woman in the Shakti position, because you have less muscle tension and greater relaxation. Many men get less vajra stimulation in this position.

Try lying on your back with your partner on top, allowing her to control the old in and out. In this position, she can support her weight relatively effortlessly by kneeling. In addition to reducing your tension and excitement, you can more easily guide your partner's motions this way. Many women like being above because it gives them maximum freedom of movement, enhancing their pleasure without the feeling of confinement underneath. Not to mention that the "superior" woman arrangement frees both partners' hands for sensual touching all over.

I know some men have a problem with what they call the "inferior" position. If you're one of them, getting used to being on the bottom will require an adjustment. If you need convincing to try it, just chalk it up to an essential step in your spiritual transformation. Remember, Male Multiple Orgasm teaches that we're each responsible for our own pleasure. Your primary concern should be on consciously surrendering to receiving pleasure, whatever the position is. If you haven't dropped that old macho thing and accepted the fact that we're all in this together to exchange ecstasy, then it's time for you to start.

A Smorgasbord of Positions

I guess I'll have to live with the judgment that I'm a rebel when I insist on disagreeing with the bulk of sexology experts. I think it's easier to learn Orgasm Mastery when you're on top. For me, I'm way more able to regulate how high I am on the 10-point arousal scale and how rapidly I peak this way.

I've learned to ride the wave when I'm on top, mostly because I get to stop, start, and make subtle adjustments. The most stimulating position for me is with my partner's legs tight together, either when I'm on top with my legs outside hers, or lying on top entering from behind.

My friend, Jay, has a different favorite position that extends lovemaking, which he calls "99." To enter 99, you engage starting from the Yab-Yum Position, with the woman sitting on your lap with both of your legs stretched out. To enter 99, simply lean back from the yab-yum position until you're both lying flat on your backs. Stroking in this position strongly rubs the top of vajra, the least sensitive surface, on your partner's G-spot.

In the final analysis, what works best for you is really up to what works best for you and your partner. Later on, I'll give you some guidelines to try all these positions so you can identify your favorites for love play.

For the time being, let's get into playing around and see what works best for you and your sweetie.

APPROACHING SLOWLY

Before you actually start thrusting, I'd like you to try several exercises that will gradually accustom vajra to yoni's stimulating energy. Partly, these slow and gentle practices are to help you relax. Partly, they are the fundamental nature of LoveMaking, slow and meditative. And partly, these exercises let you tune in to subtle orgasmic energy, your most valued partner in the Male Multiple Orgasm.

There's only one strict guideline you need to remember at all times during the coming assignments. Any respectable vajra enters a yoni only with permission. Even if you're with a long-time partner, please ask each and every time you want to visit her sacred garden.

First, we're simply going to introduce vajra to yoni and her environment without a lot of movement. This is a gentle way for vajra to acclimatize to yoni's warm, moist, and powerful energy field. Be sure you remember to breathe and find positions in which you can relax as much as possible. As you feel your energy rise, be sure to visualize it moving up your inner flute.

I won't be telling you to go all the way during these initial still exercises. Since you're a veteran of checking out what you really want in each moment, I'm guessing you can improvise whenever you choose. So, if you both prefer, by all means end these exercises with a fast-moving vajra inside yoni, enjoying him there no matter how long he lasts.

Exercise: VNY (Vajra Near Yoni)

The VNY Exercise just brings vajra near yoni. It's one of our favorite forms of foreplay at times.

You can do this whole exercise with a Shiva Lingam (an erection), but it's not necessary. If you're working with a long-time partner with whom you share unprotected sex, you can do it with a soft vajra. There are many who advocate initial yoni penetration with a softie as a normal routine. So start wherever you're at and let whatever happens happen.

You'll need to use your judgment about applying a lubricant during this exercise. It's less stimulating, of course, to do this dry. If you go too fast or use too much pressure with a partner who isn't wet, it could cause uncomfortable friction for yoni without lubrication. If you're not sure which way to go, talk about it together and decide how you want to begin. Just keep a bottle of your favorite sexual lubricant handy so you can always take a momentary break to apply more. Which, by the way, can be a welcome stop if you're getting too hot.

By the way, the final steps of this exercise suggest contact with yoni's inner lips. For this phase, you'll want to use protection with a new partner. Though the exercise is designed to acclimatize vajra, teasing yoni like this can be very exciting to your partner. If she gets really turned on, agree to pleasure her any way she wants after you clearly end the exercise.

1) Ask your partner to lie on her back with her legs spread and to stay as still as she possibly can throughout the exercise.

2) Ask your partner what kind of external lubricant she prefers, if any. Discuss when you might apply it. Have it handy before continuing.

3) Get into a Shiva or Kneeling Shiva Position between her legs with your legs extended under hers. In other words, you can also do this sitting or kneeling between her legs. Move your pelvis up close and personal to yoni. Grasp vajra's shaft with one hand, leaving the head exposed.

4) Move your hand and body to allow vajra's head to slowly and gently touch your partner's belly, hips, legs, and thighs. At first, stay away from the immediate pubic region, clio (clitoris), and yoni's lips. If you're hard enough, you can rub vajra's head and shaft anywhere he reaches. Continue this distant circling for a few minutes at least or until you feel your excitement begin to diminish. Before moving on, check in with your partner to see how she's doing and if any adjustment is needed for comfort.

5) Gradually move vajra's head closer and closer to yoni, at first lightly brushing her pubic hair.

6) Next, gently and slowly rub vajra's head in circles around yoni for a few minutes. Move up one side of the outer lips, circle above clio, slide down the outer lip on the other side, and slip across to the other side below yoni's opening.

7) Before getting any closer, reverently ask your partner's permission for vajra to approach yoni. When you're welcome, touch vajra's head to yoni's inner lips. Again, move in slow gentle circles without penetration for a few minutes. (If you've agreed to condom use, you'll need to be hard and suit up first to do this and subsequent steps. I'm sure your partner will help if you ask sweetly.)

8) Now, with permission, rub vajra's shaft up and down yoni from top to bottom in long slow strokes. Start by both of you rotating your hips forward. Place vajra's shaft on clio

lightly and ever so slowly slide vajra down until his shaft passes yoni's inner lips. Then slide up slowly. Continue this for a few minutes until you're accustomed to the excitement, increasing the pressure according to your arousal level and your partner's desire.

9) Finally, hold vajra's head in your hand. Place vajra's head lightly on clio and slide his head down between yoni's inner lips. Then move vajra's head back up again and caress clio for a few moments. Increase the pressure and speed according to your arousal level and your partner's desire.

That's all there is to getting vajra acclimated to yoni's exciting environment. If this is super exciting, you might want to repeat this exercise several times. The VNY exercise is vajra's favorite way to gear up for penetration when he starts out soft. Try rubbing vajra around yoni and clio, guiding with your hand. Invariably, he will likely get hard enough to enter yoni with a seamless transition.

Exercise: Gradual Insertion VIY

This practice is a VIY (vajra-in-yoni) version of the sensory focus exercises you did in Chapter 4. Here, you'll insert vajra slowly, relaxing, breathing, and opening your senses as widely as possible.

Initial penetration is such an exciting sexual doorway that it's one of the most difficult times to relax and enjoy. Most women love this slow, teasing, subtle approach anyway. They regard the sensitive and gentle entry (whether with your finger, tongue, or vajra) as reverent—your way of honoring the Goddess they represent.

1) Lie down together in a comfortable position and sensuously stroke each other's body while you do Orgasmic Breathing.

2) Find a comfortable sexual position for both of you where you can see both vajra and yoni. Most lovers like to begin with one on top in the Shakti or Kneeling Shiva Position. The Transverse Position is an interesting one for this exercise.

3) If you don't get hard from the sensual massage and breathing, ask your partner to pleasure vajra until you do. (Put on a condom here if agreed on.)

4) If your partner desires more stimulation before penetration, pleasure her manually, orally, or using the previous VNY exercise until she's ready. Use whatever lubrication you both prefer.

5) Ask reverently before beginning insertion. You might say *"May vajra visit your sacred garden?"*

6) Place vajra's head on yoni's inner lips. Remain there for a few moments simply feeling the energy, spreading it around your body, and letting your excitement relax. Use your breath and PC to pump the energy up.

7) Advance vajra's insertion into yoni carefully and gradually. I recommend beginning with quarter-inch increments between pauses. After each little thrust, relax, breathe, and spread the energy. Time your movements based on how long it takes your arousal to diminish. One Taoist school teaches 15 deep breaths for each inch of insertion. (If you get too excited, use Orgasmic Breathing, PC clench, perineum press, root lock, vajra squeeze, scrotal pull, or even withdrawal to avoid exploding.)

8) When vajra is completely inserted, remain still, simply feeling the sensations.

9) Stay in this position as long as possible, savoring the energetic connection. As vajra gets soft, he may remain inside or slip out. Let him do his own thing. You've learned clearly that he's got a mind of his own, right?

You may require repeated attempts to relax during Gradual Insertion without an explosive orgasm. Once you master just resting inside yoni, a whole new world of movement without a wet release opens to you.

Exercise: Karezza (Still VIY)

Karezza is a still lovemaking technique first published by Alice Bunker Stockham, a pioneering female physician, in 1883. With Karezza, vajra remains in yoni for an hour or more simply feeling the delightful energy. Whether the members of the revolutionary Oneida community in New England who developed this technique were Tantric or not, I don't know. But they sure had something that we fast-paced gratification junkies of the modern world could benefit from.

Karezza or Still VIY begins in similar fashion to the previous exercise and includes just enough movement to maintain a Shiva Lingam. The following instructions recommend that you start with the woman-on-top position, but you can actually do this any way that works best for both your bodies and arousal patterns. In any case, you'll each have a chance to move during this exercise, beginning with 10 minutes and working up to 30 each.

1) Lie down together in a comfortable position and sensuously stroke each other's body while you both do a little Orgasmic Breathing.

2) When your energy is flowing sufficiently, move into the sexual position that you found effective in the previous exercise.

3) If you don't get hard from the sensual massage and breathing, ask your partner at this point to pleasure vajra until you do. (Put on a condom here if agreed on.)

4) If your partner desires more stimulation before penetration, pleasure her manually, orally, or using the previous VNY exercise until she's ready. Use lubrication if she prefers.

5) Ask reverently before beginning insertion. You might say: *"Is your perfumed garden ready for vajra to visit?"*

6) Slowly and gradually guide vajra to enter yoni as you did in the Gradual Insertion exercise. When vajra is completely inserted, remain still, simply feeling the sensations.

7) When the excitement begins to quiet, enjoy a few shallow, leisurely thrusts. Stroke just enough to maintain a Shiva Lingam (an erect vajra). Rest as long as possible between periods of movement, feeling everything. At all times, be sure to savor as much as you can about the pleasure you're experiencing.

8) After 10 minutes of you doing the thrusting, ask your partner to do the minimum moving for 10 minutes to keep vajra hard. You'll both need to be extra conscious to communicate openly and frequently. Otherwise, she won't know how you're doing and how to adjust her motions to keep you excited at or below arousal level 9.

9) Together, decide how you want to end this exercise: continue alternating movement, withdrawing and doing something else, or really go for it.

Repeat this exercise, gradually increasing the amount of time each of you moves. Aim for 15 minutes each next time, then 20, 25, and 30. When you can each move for 30 minutes without you ejaculating, you're ready for more moving exercises.

SOME CALL IT THE OLD IN & OUT, WE CALL IT SEXUAL UNION

Cool title for this section, huh? Finally, you get to practice the old in and out. It's always been a moving experience for me.

You're far from the first person to be deeply interested in lasting longer during sexual union. There's a long history of the withdrawal technique (pulling out before ejaculating), dating from ancient Rome—where it was called *coitus reservatus*.

Actually, these exercises more closely resemble *Imsak*, a Arabic word literally meaning "retention." Imsak obviously refers to retaining your semen inside while making love. Imsak was apparently developed for men who needed to satisfy an entire harem each night and couldn't keep getting it up again and again with each lover.

Most experts advise the following sequence of the next two exercises: In the first, you stay still inside yoni while she moves. In the second, your partner stays still, demonstrating extreme loving patience, while you do the motions. I have to admit that I'm not really sure about which order will be best for you. The opposite order works better for me, where first I get to control sexual thrusting motions instead of depending on communication with my partner to avoid getting too excited. Read them both and decide with your partner which you want to do first.

Even though I haven't instructed you each time, you've been remembering to relax and breathe during all practices, right? In the same way, to save time, I'm not going to precede each exercise with directions to get comfortable, exchange foreplay, get vajra hard, and put on a condom if you've agreed to. You'll remember to do that during all your LoveMaking practices, won't you?

Exercise: Still Stop-Start VIY

Yeah, that's a funny title for this exercise. It means you remain still while your partner gets to move, stopping and starting according to your directions. Since you're very familiar with this drill in other settings, the peaking cycle should come naturally. By the way, it's great to continue kissing and sensual touching all over your partner's body when you pause between motions. Many lovers like this kind of variation during lovemaking and appreciate the attention to the entire body.

1) After preliminaries, get into whatever position you prefer.

2) Ask if she is ready for vajra and guide him to slowly penetrate yoni.

3) When vajra is completely inserted, remain still, simply feeling the sensations until your excitement begins to lessen.

4) Ask your partner to begin moving while you remain still.

5) Be sure to communicate openly and frequently so she knows how you're doing and how to adjust her motions. Guide her using the feedback sandwich to vary how fast, deep, and energetically yoni bounces on vajra.

6) When you peak at arousal level 6, signal your partner to stop moving completely. Take a deep breath, hold it, and squeeze your PC muscle until you drop down a couple levels. You know the drill well, by now.

7) Repeat peaking at arousal level 6 five more times using stop-starts.

8) In the same way, peak at arousal levels 8 and 9, six times each.

Repeat this practice as many times as you need until you can last for 30 minutes without an explosive orgasm. Of course, the more implosive ones you have the better. The more you do Still Stop-Start VIY, and the closer you get to the point-of-no return without going over the edge while being relaxed, the more you're likely to experience dry orgasms (contractions without ejaculating). Enjoy!

Exercise: Moving Stop-Start VIY

Now you get to switch roles. Your partner stays still and you move, using stop-start. Because vajra's corona and frenulum are very sensitive, some find the least stimulating place to stop is pressing into yoni as deeply as possible. Some find the opposite true. Test it out and learn what works best for you.

As you begin developing your skill, you may need to withdraw vajra partly or completely to manage your arousal level. You can even switch to pleasuring your partner with your fingers or mouth during short breaks as you recover.

You've obviously perfected your signals and communication skills by this point. Just a reminder: during this drill, don't stop moving inside without explanation. Of course, some day you may discover that you're totally in sync with each other, tele-pathically knowing exactly what's going on inside your partner. Until you reach that mystical arena, keep communicating. Otherwise, you can create mutual tension, which we all know contributes to an involuntary wet release.

1) Lie on your back with your partner straddling you. Or if you find you can regulate your movements easier from above, get on top of your partner.

2) Ask if she is ready for vajra and guide him to slowly pene-trate yoni. When vajra is completely inserted, remain still, simply feeling the sensations until your excitement begins to lessen.

3) Ask your partner to remain still while you begin moving.

4) Keep communicating openly and frequently about what's going on inside you.

5) When you peak at arousal level 6, signal your partner and stop moving completely. Take a deep breath, hold it, and squeeze your PC muscle until you drop down a cou-ple levels. Old hat, right?

6) Repeat peaking at arousal level 6 five more times using stop-starts.

7) In the same way, peak at arousal levels 8 and 9 six times each.

Repeat this practice as many times as you need until you can last for 30 minutes without losing it.

Exercise: Both Moving Stop-Start VIY

You've got more to practice to completely master the Male Multiple Orgasm. But you've come so far! Now you get to experi-ence both you and your partner moving while making love.

I probably don't have to mention it, but let me remind you that letting go with wild abandon may still cause a quick explo-sive orgasm. This exercise is a slow, sensuous, measured climb up the arousal scale. OK, now that I've preached a bit, I'll let you in on a secret.

Tantric adepts are known far and wide for their ability to please women. These "experts" make love in a manner that closely resembles how this exercise unfolds. They don't pump strenuously and continuously until their partner orgasms. Instead, they tease, tickle, and tantalize for the longest time. Instead of succumbing to the urge to ejaculate that still makes an unexpected occurrence, they dance with their own energy and the rising tide of ecstasy in their partner. They're not rushing headlong toward the goal of the Big O. No, they're savoring every little sensation themselves and milking the interplay for all the pleasure it's worth.

You're learning how to do that very thing. Don't blow it now. Just keep floating in that endless sea of orgasmic energy without consciously causing the explosion. Sometimes it will visit unannounced of its own accord. When it does, surrender and let it sweep both of you away together.

1) After preliminaries, get into whatever position you prefer.

2) Ask if she is ready for vajra and guide him to slowly penetrate yoni. When vajra is completely inserted, remain still, simply feeling the sensations until your excitement begins to lessen.

3) Ask your partner to move slowly, while you move as well.

4) Both of you should keep communicating openly and frequently about what's going on inside each of you.

5) When you peak at arousal level 6, signal your partner and both stop moving completely. Take a deep breath, hold it, and squeeze your PC muscle until you drop down a couple levels.

6) Repeat peaking at arousal level 6 five more times using stop-starts.

7) In the same way, peak at 8 and 9 six times each.

Repeat this practice as many times as you need until you can last for 30 minutes without a wet release.

DANCING WITH SEXUAL UNION: THE ART OF FUCKING

Yes, my titles are getting more and more descriptive. Why not consider how you move vajra in and out of yoni an art?

As your love stamina increases, a whole range of possibilities opens up to you. You can always resort to fast animal pumping when you really want to. But let's put our attention on S.E.X., Subtle Energy eXchange, and create a spiritual merger instead of an Olympic strength event.

The final exercises in Chapter 7 are about extending your growing skill to more closely resemble spontaneous lovemaking without structure. Instead of stop-start, we'll now use the familiar subtle adjustments to peak and plateau, followed by Orgasmic Breathing to channel energy up and away from your hot spots. As well, I'll suggest some different sexual positions to play with.

Exercise: Subtle Adjustments VIY

Subtle Adjustments VIY begins just like the previous exercise, in which you both moved and stopped when necessary to avoid slipping past 9.9. Here, you'll use subtle adjustments to get your excitement level to back off. Of course, those changes are different when you're inside yoni and not using a hand or two.

For example, while you're underneath on your back, you can slide your body up toward your partner's head. Then the angle of vajra's entry will be more perpendicular to the bed instead of toward your lover's head. The advantage of this higher angle of entry is that there's less friction on vajra's more sensitive underside. Women like this because it increases stimulation on clio (their clitoris).

Or you can shift from straight in-and-out strokes to circular or side-to-side rocking motions. For many men, these strokes provide less stimulation to vajra's sensitive head. Circular strokes can rub clio with your lower belly or grind your pubic bone on your partner's.

Another way to lessen your excitement while inside yoni is to use shallower strokes. Not only do shorter thrusts tantalize many women, but moving less without completely withdrawing can help you last longer. Since the outer third of yoni is more sensitive, many women prefer these shallower vajra motions. Further, shallower thrusts excite clio by pulling more on yoni's outer walls.

The tantalizing effect of these adjustments provides more evidence that deep fast pumping may not be the most stimulating for many women. Why hump away nonstop and make yourself explode quickly just because of some porno-flick-inspired fantasy?

1) After preliminaries, get into whatever sexual position works best for you.

2) Ask if your partner is ready for vajra and guide him to slowly penetrate yoni. When vajra is completely inserted, remain still, simply feeling the sensations until your excitement begins to lessen.

3) Ask your partner to move slowly while you move as well.

4) Both of you should keep communicating openly and frequently about what's going on inside each of you.

5) When you reach arousal level 6, instead of stopping, vary what you're doing to reduce the excitement a few points (for example, down to arousal level 4). Slow down, change position and direction, thrust more shallowly, or lighten the pressure of your strokes. Peak like this six times.

6) Repeat subtle adjustment peaking six times at arousal level 8, and then at 9.

7) Now, use subtle adjustments to plateau, first at arousal level 6, then 8, and then 9, or higher.

If you want greater structure, try the Taoist 9 and 1 technique. Taoist sexual texts recommend that men use more shallow strokes than deep ones to retain their semen while exciting their lovers. Thrust according to the following regimen:

3 shallow, then 1 deep—repeat 81 times

5 shallow, then 1 deep—repeat 81 times

9 shallow, then 1 deep—repeat 81 times

As you develop more and more mastery, the Taoists suggest you repeat this sequence with 2 deep thrusts, instead of 1, and then with 3 deep thrusts, instead of 1, and using vajra's entire length.

When you can regulate your excitement level subtly, what's to keep you from going forever? You're really getting close to graduating now. Just a few more titillating variations ahead.

Exercise: Orgasmic Breathing VIY

As you've done before with self-pleasuring, your next assignment is to use Orgasmic Breathing to channel the energy throughout your body.

1) After preliminaries, get into whatever sexual position works best for you.

2) Ask if she is ready for vajra and guide him to slowly penetrate yoni. When vajra is completely inserted, remain still, simply feeling the sensations until your excitement begins to lessen.

3) Ask your partner to move slowly while you move as well.

4) Both of you should keep communicating openly and frequently about what's going on inside each of you.

5) When you reach arousal level 6, instead of stopping, slow down slightly. Open your eyes wide, inhale more deeply into the belly, but this time through the NOSE, and hold

your breath. Relax completely as you exhale, visualizing your sexual fire streaming out of vajra, and moaning with pleasure to release energy.

6) Inhale again through the nose, visualizing that pleasurable energy moving up vajra through your pelvis to your heart and higher. Use one long or several short PC Pumps to help you shoot the energy upward. Peak like this six times.

7) Repeat peaking using Orgasmic Breathing six times at arousal level 8 and then at 9.

8) Now, use Orgasmic Breathing to plateau, first at arousal level 6, then 8, and then 9, or higher.

As you get more comfortable with your ability to maintain a high level of excitement, you'll be able to float closer and closer to 9.9. The more you relax and open to orgasmic energy, the more you'll experience implosive orgasms. You will find that, as you learn to handle more and more energy, your point of no return gets higher and higher.

Exercise: Different Positions

If you're like me and most other guys, you've found your preferred sexual position and used it for these exercises. That's fine. If you haven't, I applaud you for moving ahead at your own pace. Regardless, it's time to play with the other sexual positions available to adventuresome students like yourself. This exercise will be more freeform than previous ones. As you experiment, use everything here that works for you.

Below, I've listed multiple variations of the seven basic sexual postures. What's the best order for experimenting? There's no scientific standard, so pay your money and take your chances.

You remember the old joke about the octogenarian at a sex lecture who yelled from the back row that he'd tried 101 postures. After the laughter died down and the speaker started describing the missionary position, the geezer jumped up screaming "102, 102!" Well, I probably haven't covered every position here, and certainly haven't detailed the exact arrangement of your limbs in each case. This exercise is included to stretch your comfort zone around postures you might not otherwise experiment with. With perseverance and a little luck, you just might find combinations that turn your partner on while maintaining your excitement at a manageable level.

As you try out different postures, keep your attention focused on your arousal and your sexual energy. Which positions turn both of you on the most? Which strokes please you both the most in which positions? In which postures can you relax the most? In which positions can you sexually breathe—rock your pelvis, breathe in the belly, squeeze your PC—with most effect? Which postures allow your energy to flow up your inner flute the most?

Dozens of Tantric LoveMaking Postures

You can modify each of the seven basic *Kama Sutra* positions by moving torsos, adjusting limbs, and changing how you support yourselves. To bring some order to all the options, I've grouped the variations of each position into several categories that I call *postures*. In addition, each posture can be changed into numerous variations by shifting arms, legs, and body weight.

The following list offers several postures for each of the seven positions:

Shakti Position (Woman on Top, You're on Your Back)
> **Kneeling Forward:** she kneels over, facing your head.
> **Squatting Forward:** she squats over, facing your head.
> **Lying Forward:** she lies forward, facing your head.
> **Sitting on Top:** she sits on top of you.
> **Facing Backward:** she faces your feet.

We've discussed some pros and cons of the Shakti Position. There's less stress on you on the bottom, but regulating your peaks and plateaus depends on communication, coordination, and how synchronized you are. Some of these postures are tighter than others, which seems to have the greatest impact on staying power. Some of the angles of penetration, like Sitting On Top and Lying Forward, can be more stimulating than others.

Shiva Position (Man on Top, Woman on Back)

Her Legs Together: her legs are together.

Flanquette: she's half-facing you.

Her Legs Wide: her thighs are wide, you're between her legs.

Her Legs Up: her legs are high.

Again, in the Shiva Position, where your legs are influences the tightness and angle of penetration more than anything else. How high you ride can influence whether vajra's most sensitive parts get the most friction. Wide legs are less arousing than legs together.

Kneeling Shiva Position (She's on Her Back, You're Between Her Legs)

Wide Open: her body is raised up.

Holding: she holds you tight.

Chest: her feet are on your chest.

Shoulders: her feet are on your shoulders.

Head: her feet are on your head.

These are simply further extensions of the Shiva Position. Wide Open is usually the least stimulating, while the variations with her legs up tend to be tighter and more arousing.

Transverse Position (Side-to-Side)

Woman on Back: she's on her back, you're at right angles to her.

Woman on Side: she's on her side, you kneel behind her.

Both on Sides: you face each other, both on your sides.

Depending on the arrangement of your intersecting legs, you can make Transverse Postures tight or loose. A primary advantage of side-to-side positions is that the man can vary his thrusting without the effort of supporting himself. Also, all four hands are free for other stimulation.

Cow Position (Rear Entry)

Bent Over: she's bent over with you behind her.
Face Down: she lies face down, you're on top.
Sideways: she's on her side, you're behind her.

Rear entry positions are often some of the most exciting. Maybe that's because your partner's legs are closer together, creating more friction on vajra's sides. Bent Over, the classic doggie position, allows for quite a bit of variation, while Face Down tends to be the tightest. The disadvantage of these positions is that communication is more difficult, since you can't maintain eye contact.

Yab-Yum Position (Sitting)

Yab-Yum: you sit cross-legged with her on your lap.
Straddling: you straddle one another with one or more legs.
Raised: you sit cross-legged, she's on your lap with legs raised.
Leaning: from *yab-yum* both lean back partway.
Further Back: from *yab-yum* both lean back to the floor.

Sitting Positions are exciting but vajra's stimulation often depends on the relative sizes of your jewels and strength of both your PC muscles. These facing positions are some of the most demanding physically but satisfying energetically. By facing each other, it's easier to align your chakras and channel your energy upward. The delight of Yab-Yum, the classic Tantric LoveMaking position, provides great motivation to go to the gym regularly or develop greater flexibility with Yoga postures. Speaking of which, some of these positions are much easier when sitting on a hard meditation pillow like a Japanese *zafu*.

Both Standing: both stand.

Suspended: she's suspended from your body.

Bed or Table: she lies on her back, you stand between her legs.

Love Swing: she lies in a hammock, you stand between her legs.

These unusual *Kama Sutra* postures can be fun but demanding, especially when you're both standing. As before, wideness versus looseness and angle of entry have the biggest impact on vajra's sensitivity.

With such a wide spectrum of possibilities, I guess you can see that there are lots of factors under your control that can influence tightness and the arousal from stroking. You see there's a lot of arduous practice ahead of you...

1) Discuss which positions you want to try before you begin making love.

2) After sensuous touching, move into the first position you selected and, with permission, insert vajra into yoni.

3) Slowly move together, monitoring your arousal level, peaking several times at arousal levels 6, 8, and 9.

4) If you find this posture too arousing, use stop-start, subtle adjustments, and Orgasmic Breathing or even ejaculation interruption techniques to avoid going over the top.

5) Try other positions, peaking at increasing levels several times.

6) When you find a position that's exciting for both of you, play with plateauing as long as you like.

7) Is it time to go for simultaneous orgasm? You decide.

Don't try to practice with every position and posture during one lovemaking session. Repeat this exercise, trying several postures at a time. When you've explored them all, you'll know what you prefer. For variety, try various positions at different times.

Congratulations on your advanced skills. By arriving at this point in the Male Multiple Orgasm practice program, you've changed your skills and patterns tremendously. Now, at last, you have the credentials to qualify for the secret rites of Male Multiple Orgasm LoveMaking (most of which you've already figured out, I bet).

POP QUIZ

Here's your ticket to moving on. Answer the following questions honestly:

1) Do you still sometimes feel a strong urge to ejaculate?
2) Do you fight it or beat yourself up about it?
3) Do you know how to direct the energy that's causing this urge upward and inward without always exploding outward?
4) Are you ready for dancing with all you know in the altered space of continuous rapture?

Now let's score your test.

- If you answered yes to (1), score 1 point. If you answered no, it's hard for me to believe, but score 2 points with gusto.
- If you answered yes to (2), you need to practice releasing your inner struggles more. You get 1 point for knowing yourself and answering honestly. If you answered no, well, again it's hard to believe but score 2 points.
- If you answered yes to (3), score 1 point. If you answered no, score 1 point for honesty. But I strongly suggest you go back and practice more before continuing.

Regardless of your answers to (1) through (3), your answer to (4) determines whether you're ready to move on to Chapter 8. Yes, they were all trick questions. Would you expect any less from me after all we've been through together?

CHAPTER 8

✧ *Orgasmic Energy Mastery*

Welcome, my friend, to Orgasmic Energy Mastery. By arriving here, you've developed all the faculties needed to put Male Multiple Orgasm (MMO) into action whenever you make love.

This chapter is all about the last R of RAMPER, which is Ride the wave. It's a wave of orgasmic energy, of love bliss, of ecstatic delirium, of spiritual rapture. Once you experience it fully, it will certainly transform your lovemaking, your relationship, and maybe even your whole life.

In the earlier chapters, you've experimented with—and hopefully perfected—a wide spectrum of new skills to help you enjoy MMO. Chapter 8 simply brings all the pieces together into what I call an entirely new sexual style: Orgasmic Energy LovePlay, or just Energy LovePlay, for short.

It's only fair for me to warn you at this point that you won't be satisfied with ordinary sex driven by pure animal lust anymore. When you taste your connection to the divine through Orgasmic Energy LovePlay, you'll want to stay there, at home spiritually, basking in the mindless serenity. Sorry, sometimes I get carried away waxing poetic while trying to describe this indescribable experience.

Though by now you're no stranger to Orgasmic Energy Mastery, in Chapter 8 I'm going to sum up all its fundamental principles in one place. Then I'll compare Energy LovePlay with everyday garden-variety sex, and then remind you how to use the tools you've learned.

There are only two practices in this chapter: creating the space for Energy LovePlay, and experiencing it. I call the last one the Shangri-La exercise. There's little doubt that you'll want to do these again and again.

THE PRINCIPLES OF ORGASMIC ENERGY MASTERY

As you gain Orgasmic Energy Mastery, you'll become a highly skilled lover who can give enormous pleasure and enjoy MMO at will. But you'll find that your learning curve won't be purely defined by skillful sexual techniques. Your sexual style will become more like meditation than an athletic sport. That's because, as you follow the ebb and flow of orgasmic energy, you'll play without set patterns, without expectations, and without measurable goals.

You won't rush through foreplay to get to the main act and judge success in the sack by making your partner climax. Instead, you'll focus on S.E.X., which means Subtle Energy eXchange. Ultimately, you'll discover that S.E.X. is any touch, motion, or exchange that connects your inner vibrations with your lover's to create pinnacles of pleasure for both of you. You see, you'll be operating on a much more expanded plane than just the genital friction of sexual union.

Here are the principles that allow you to enjoy this kind of Energy LovePlay to the max. The more you take them into your mind, body, and spirit, the more you'll ascend to this heavenly style of sex.

Wake Up and Smell the Roses

So many people are swept through life looking at pictures in the mind instead of living moment to moment. They spend their consciousness dwelling on the past, plotting the future, and comparing the current state of affairs to a set of prerecorded subconscious tapes. This kind of mental condition doesn't reinforce the Orgasmic Energy Mastery you need for male multiple orgasm.

To counteract this programming, Energy LovePlay requires you to pay more attention and focus your mind on the present. It teaches you to be supremely conscious of everything that happens while you watch and enjoy. When you learn to exist in this moment and become totally absorbed in the "now," you open your windows to the world fully. You do this by heightening your five senses: sight, smell, taste, touch, and hearing. You become dedicated to enjoying the physical fully by reveling in eating, drinking, massaging, dancing, and making love.

But even more, I'm talking about knowing yourself and the world around you as more than just a material shell. Complete honesty and authenticity about your truth is essential for the kind of spiritual growth that Energy LovePlay activates. As you learn to observe yourself, accept the wisdom of your heart, and shine bright light on your inner knowing, you discover a clearer idea of your deeper self—of who you really are.

If you get to know yourself better, will the truth really set you free? What will you find underneath all those layers of old baggage hiding the real inner self?

Your Natural Self

A fundamental underpinning of Orgasmic Energy Mastery is that your essential make-up is love and that your true nature is blissful. Inside you is a spontaneous, joyous, playful, childlike spirit who wants to be free to savor everything and love everyone. As a result, it's only natural you would honor sex as a celebration of life and have a desire to merge your soul with another.

So why don't most of us behave that way if that's our basic nature? Modern Western upbringing doesn't teach these underlying values of self-love and enjoyment of life. Instead, we're made unnatural by social conditioning and by moral codes that don't serve our inherent make-up. All these dos and don'ts produce inner struggles against our basic desires.

What can you do about your upbringing? You can be conscious of who you are and what you want. Recognize which desires spring from your inner being and which have been impressed on you. Don't resist healthy impulses, which would inhibit your vital spirit from emerging if you denied them. Shed the social conventions that bring you down and release the brainwashing that doesn't serve you. If you follow an impulse that's not part of your essential nature, you learn from these experiments to drop it. If you find great satisfaction in what you pursue, you can only conclude that you've discovered more of your personal truth.

Welcome Your Other Side

The fuel that drives Male Multiple Orgasm stems in large part from your masculinity. Whether it's the primal urge to propagate the species or the drive to conquer the "weaker sex," letting your male nature flow is essential to excelling at Orgasmic Energy Mastery. Yet to do that, instead of fighting and controlling, you have to relax, accept, and surrender to these powerful life forces. That kind of behavior is decidedly feminine.

Western society artificially separates people's inner masculine and feminine qualities by discouraging their development. Men are taught, for example, to hide their femininity. Energy LovePlay requires each gender to cultivate the latent energies of the other.

If men seek their intrinsic truths on this path, they'll invariably discover their soft, receptive, sensitive, and vulnerable side without losing their masculinity. Women will discover their strong leadership, dynamic initiative, and teaching powers while retaining their femininity. These qualities will only add to the strengths consistent with your outer gender, which you've already learned to exercise.

Here's a simple formula for awakening your inner femininity without sacrificing your virility. Instead of creating a picture of how you're supposed to be, operate on the principle that the way out is the way through. Fully confront the joys and stresses that come your way. Above all else, relax and go with the flow, allowing your innate forces to run their course. Watch and learn and discover that the truth will set you free.

It Takes a Real Man to Practice Surrender

To fully embrace Orgasmic Energy Mastery, you need to say YES! to life. Accept everything and forbid nothing. Drop moral judgments about right and wrong or good and bad. Instead, come from a place of wholeness, embracing opposites as aspects of the same thing. Recognize that judgments like good and bad are based on artificial yardsticks held fast in your subconscious mind. To cast off this programming, learn to live in harmony with whatever life serves up, whether on a silver platter or bed of thorns. Learn the New Age practice of surrender, which means just letting things happen of their own accord without resistance.

Give up the intoxicating illusion that you can and should control everything in the outside world.

Essential to practicing Male Multiple Orgasm is accepting that if you suppress natural inner forces, they won't disappear, they'll just fester and then insinuate their way to the surface in an unhealthy manner. Orgasmic Energy Mastery teaches you to embrace all parts of yourself and everything that befalls you. If you don't buy others' moral codes that conflict you, what's there to hide? If there's no good and bad, why not just drop guilt? If there's no right or wrong, why not release all shame? If everything in life is divine, what's there to fear? If God is love, why can't you experience heaven on earth?

To major in surrender and let the energy flow, don't fight, resist, or reject things. That kind of personal suppression can only produce mental warfare and internal stress. Release all stress as a useless struggle with no winners, only losers. Let go of the futile attempt to stop things that are happening from happening. Maybe that's what Paul McCartney was singing about in "Let It Be."

As a result, you have to learn to accept constant change. What's right for you now may not be the next moment. And vice versa. What's right for others—no matter how much we envy them—may be wrong for you. And vice versa. How could you follow prescribed patterns if you're responding to life genuinely in every unique moment? All you can do is risk, explore, observe, listen, and notice, choosing what brings you joy and growth and leaving the rest behind.

This whole approach to life suggests you should just give up goal orientation, enter each experience without expectations, and just live fully in each moment. But to love life and others requires that you accept one fundamental truth: even with all your judgments about your shortcomings, you're perfect the way you are. You're never going to arrive at some imagined state of perfection. Your journey is just exactly the way it needs to be.

Honor the Body Temple

The key to joyous living is first loving yourself. This begins with an exceedingly difficult assignment: accepting your body the way it is now. I'm not just referring to your height, weight, and looks. It's rare for a guy in the modern world not to be concerned about vajra's size, stamina, and staying power.

The media and mass consciousness, having created the vision of the perfect form, encourages you to fill yourself full of negative judgments about your anatomy. Orgasmic Energy Mastery demands that you not to fall for these false standards but, instead, cherish your body as the temple of your soul.

While it's true that most major religions view the pleasures of the flesh as degraded or evil, you need to release that outmoded programming to fully experience MMO. Recognize that your physical form is a divine gift—one that houses your spirit and lets your inner being experience the sights, sounds, and smells of the physical world. Regardless of its size, shape, or color, your body deserves your unconditional love and affection just for letting you delight in so many delicious sensations. Further, it helps you think, communicate, move, and act.

Face it, sex wouldn't be much fun at all without a body. Don't you think life would be much duller if you were just a disembodied spirit?

Put Pleasure First

Orgasmic Energy Mastery only comes at a price, and that price is committing yourself to enjoying life to the fullest. OK, at first, that doesn't seem like much of a sacrifice.

But cultural programming for deferred gratification—be good, follow the rules, and you'll earn your ticket to heaven in the next life—makes fully embracing pleasure a real challenge.

As a practitioner of Male Multiple Orgasm, you've got to believe in enjoying life to the fullest. The true art of living and loving this way makes pleasure the central theme in each moment.

To make this work, you'll probably need a shift in priorities. You have to put pleasure first and make space in your busy life to appreciate, enjoy, and be happy.

This isn't as easy as it sounds. It requires more than just reserving playtime in your overstuffed calendar. You've got to learn to cultivate ecstasy, to surrender to sensation, and to pursue pleasure with gusto. Just when you start feeling good, your conditioning might kick in, making you feel that you're being selfish, having too much fun, or don't deserve it. You've got to unlearn the guilt and resistance that's bred into you. Your body needs to learn that pleasure is its birthright.

In other words, make pleasure a discipline. Teach yourself to increase your capacity to enjoy, accept more and more sensation, and value it more through Energy LovePlay.

THE HEALING POWER
OF ENERGY LOVEPLAY

Through conscious practice of Male Multiple Orgasm techniques, you will become a better lover. Your erections will become stronger, you'll make love longer, and experience bigger and better prolonged orgasms. Your experience will deepen and open up new levels of intimate communion. Along the way, you'll heal your wounds, lose your inhibitions, and release your inner blocks by seeking higher and higher states of ecstasy.

Male Multiple Orgasm wasn't designed as therapy for your sexual hang-ups and limitations, it just sometimes turns out that way. When you relax, exercise your erogenous zones, and enjoy your body, you might well run into the old baggage that blocks your excitement. You could discover that old pains, wounds, and trauma are stored in your tissues.

But instead of focusing on problems, Orgasmic Energy LovePlay heals purely through the committed pursuit of pleasure. By opening your energy channels, you'll work through any resistance that surfaces. You'll be left cleansed, relaxed, and free.

Drop Any Judgments

Too many lovers judge their partners according to some hidden inner picture of the perfect man or woman. Unconsciously, we create scenarios in our mind, project certain behavior, and then judge harshly when what we expect doesn't happen. Sometimes we don't like what our playmate is doing, but all too often it's ourselves that we give a devastating report card.

Projecting, expecting, and judging don't work well in the world of orgasmic energy because Energy LovePlay only flows without an agenda. It's all about feeling pleasure, nothing more and nothing less, in each moment. When you do this, criticism disappears along with any mystery about what's happening with your partner. Performance anxiety (Am I doing it right?) gets replaced with a sense of welcoming and enjoying the unexpected.

You might compare Orgasmic Energy LovePlay to one-on-one synchronized swimming with telepathic communication.

To play with orgasmic energy, you must continuously be responsible for your own pleasure in each moment. Recognize that erotic experiences begin WITHIN. Be aware of what you like, what you want right now, and what you prefer to leave out of this encounter.

Obviously, this kind of authentic interplay requires knowing, accepting, and loving yourself fully first. Then you can be scrupulously honest, totally real, and refreshingly transparent with your innermost desires—which leads to knowing, accepting, and loving your beloved.

Stay in Instant Communication

The only way that Orgasmic Energy LovePlay can work is if you ask for what you want, voice your reactions, and give lots of feedback. And do it in a way that enhances intimacy and contributes to the sensual mood. That's why playing with Orgasmic Energy together absolutely requires staying in instant communication with your partner.

ENERGY IS LIFE FORCE

As you well know by now, Male Multiple Orgasm is about mastering energy, the vitality of life. Everything in the physical universe is in motion due to energy flowing. The cells in your body, the blood in your veins, the electrical impulses in your nerves all continuously vibrate inside.

Energy is the physical oscillations that your body feels all the time. If not for feeling energy moving, how would you become aware of being turned on, angry, nervous, or in love? You feel energetic sensations in your body: the heat that spreads in waves, the arousal that raises goose bumps, the tingles and tickles that titillate.

During Energy LovePlay, you're working with the nervous stimulation and physical excitation that causes these feelings. Since the strongest energy most people experience is just before an orgasm, I call it orgasmic energy in exercises and rituals. But it's all the same electrical and magnetic life force in your body.

Orgasmic Energy Mastery requires heightened awareness of these subtler, finer frequencies. Most people don't notice them because their receivers haven't been tuned to pick them up. But when you do, there's so much delight in exploring your senses of taste, sight, smell, and sound as well as deeper appreciation of sensual touch. Because energy flows where attention goes, your consciousness becomes your most powerful energy-focusing tool. As you learn to harness these subtle vibrations—guiding the flows, channeling the energy—it ultimately creates powerful tidal waves of ecstasy.

In China, it's called chi; in India, it's called prana; in Japan, it's called ki—but it's all energy. I'm talking about the same life force that pervades body, mind, and soul. You've learned that energy is generated and stored in each of your seven chakras. Remember, chakras are centers or vortices inside the body, from the bottom of the spine to the top of the head, where subtle energy is generated, collected, and stored. At each center, the energy swirls with different qualities.

Ecstasy Orgasm

We all build up sexual tension in our bodies. Consequently, untrained lovers too often treat sex as a way to relieve this pressure and blow off steam. These mini-explosions release energy quickly in a few-second flash of pleasure. There's nothing wrong with a hot quickie now and then. But explosive orgasm, more so for men when accompanied by ejaculation, often drains lovers of their vital essence.

Most untrained lovers' orgasms are more like a little sneeze than fireworks moving heaven and earth. In Energy LovePlay, orgasm becomes a much different experience. It becomes a sacred energy event, separate from energy release and physical ejaculation. Instead of throwing it away in a quick burst, you learn to utilize and recycle sexual energy as the raw material that creates divine ecstasy and higher consciousness.

Through Orgasmic Energy Mastery, you cultivate the ecstatic response, which you might call an orgasm inside your nervous system. By conserving and channeling orgasmic energy within, you experience long-lasting implosive orgasms. Instead of discharging, the energy implodes, flooding the entire body with pulsing orgasmic contractions and continuous wavelike vibrations. You shake all over, engulfed in surge after surge of pure liquid fire. Because you're conserving sexual energy instead of expending it, these streams of ecstasy can go on and on and higher and higher. In fact, adepts in Orgasmic Energy Mastery can generate and flow this energy without sexual stimulation.

In these glimpses of a higher dimension, you enter a timeless void and seem to become one with the universe. You feel your body, mind, and spirit merging with your beloved. You enter an altered state of awareness. In this rapture, it seems as if your physical limitations disappear and you float with all boundaries dissolved. Suddenly, you're open to flowing pure positive energy from your innate blissful source. You become a conduit for communion between earth and sky, the physical and the spiritual.

Achieving this state is really the ultimate focus of Male Multiple Orgasm practice. You learn to find true ecstasy within by relaxing into high states of arousal. You channel the life force that sexuality generates and expand the energy up your inner flute, the subtle pathway that connects your chakras. You weave the essence of all your centers—body, mind, spirit—into holistic union with all that is. This is true bliss, being at one with the universe.

Sex as Meditation

Maybe that's why those who revel in Orgasmic Energy LovePlay sometimes describe sex as meditation. Meditation is simply sitting and emptying the mind. Since you can't force thoughts away, this is more challenging than it sounds. Over the millennia, gurus have developed many meditation techniques, from reciting mantras to watching the breath to witnessing ideas floating by. They all seek to create a deep inner peace filled with stillness. We call this presence a "no mind" condition.

When you cultivate the continuous state of inner orgasm, you'll naturally find yourself drawn to this meditative state. To encourage the no-mind condition, Energy LovePlay begins with ritual to prepare your mind and body for complete relaxation. You enter this kind of lovemaking without goals or expectations, surrendering to whatever unfolds. All of this creates the non-resistant mood in which you can consciously summon energy to flow.

ORGASMIC ENERGY LOVEPLAY

If you took a snapshot of Orgasmic Energy LovePlay, at any given moment it might look a lot like ordinary sex. Yet it ultimately unfolds much differently than the average quickie hurtling downhill to explosive release. It's slow, spontaneous, and conscious. It's open, intimate, and mutual. It more closely resembles a team sport like soccer or basketball than individual performances such as gymnastics or sprint swimming.

Comparing Ordinary Sex to Orgasmic Energy LovePlay

Orgasmic Energy LovePlay is more like sensuously sipping an expensive Cabernet than chugging a six-pack of brew. It more resembles sampling the delicacies at a gourmet buffet than inhaling a pepperoni pizza during Monday Night Football. It's certainly more like a twilight stroll through a perfumed garden during spring with your beloved on your arm than running a hundred-yard dash.

Energy LovePlay is leisurely, savoring every delicious morsel of pleasure, instead of rushing headlong toward maximum turn-on now. Lovers who concentrate on orgasmic energy often move ever so slowly, stopping frequently to settle deeply into the rising tide of pleasure, stretching the experience out as long as possible. Releasing tension and giving in to the urge to explode is replaced with continuous streaming vibrations of ecstatic energy. When you enter the altered state of consciousness that comes with repeated implosive orgasms, you simply want to float upon a cloud of bliss together.

Don't get me wrong, all kinds of sex are great. Remember, we define S.E.X. as Subtle Energy eXchange. In the enlightened view, any consenting sex is good sex. That could simply be sensuous massage, sharing mental fantasies, or a juicy quickie. So when I extol the celestial virtues of Energy LovePlay, don't think that I mean to judge other kinds of play negatively. It's just another option that opens to the MMO adept, albeit a fantastic one.

Let's compare Ordinary Sex with Energy LovePlay in detail:

- Ordinary Sex is a purely physical event with the goal of releasing tension and semen. Energy LovePlay is a spiritual meditation focused on continuing pleasure.
- Ordinary Sex rushes headlong toward an explosive orgasm. Energy LovePlay generates multiple continuous, full-body, implosive orgasms that can culminate in an earth-shattering simultaneous explosion.
- Ordinary Sex targets the jewels, building and releasing energy quickly in one explosive peak. Energy LovePlay awakens the whole body slowly, moving energy up the chakras to reach higher and higher plateaus and energize the spiritual centers.
- Ordinary Sex begins with goals and expectations, often creating frustration and performance anxiety. Energy

LovePlay is spontaneous, without pattern, responding to the whims of the moment.

- Ordinary Sex is often quiet, with fast, shallow breathing. Energy LovePlay is verbal, noisy, and stimulated by slow deep belly breathing.
- Ordinary Sex is tense, often closed and private, and requires fast pumping to avoid losing the mood or the erection. Energy LovePlay is relaxed, open, varied, often starting and stopping as a result of intimate communication.
- Ordinary Sex depends on one lover getting the other off. Energy LovePlay depends on each lover's skill in taking responsibility for their own pleasure.
- Ordinary Sex doesn't happen without an erection, the loss of which is a major calamity. Energy LovePlay uses multiple hard and soft stimulators on many erogenous zones, all of which are capable of producing orgasmic waves of energy with or without an erection.
- Ordinary Sex unexpectedly reaches heights of passion on occasion due to unknown factors. Energy LovePlay can generate altered states of ecstatic consciousness almost at will.

Moving Energy

How do you reach such mind-boggling heights? Simple: By generating and channeling orgasmic energy. The biological forces of sex certainly produce lots of energy in your jewels, especially when you're young and healthy. But what happens when you age or get stressed by sickness or life pressures? Then you can't depend on hormones to turn you on and make you high. You have to master running energy.

Orgasmic Breathing is the key to running orgasmic energy. Relaxing, breathing, moving, making sounds, and focusing the mind are its essential tools. That's partly why I've been including breathing exercises at each stage of Male Multiple Orgasm. Like any new skill, you need to practice regularly to integrate this vital method into your sexual encounters.

That reminds me of an early session in my personal, year-long training in the mid-1990s. My teacher was presenting another sexual practice in her frank and flamboyant style. As she graphically described how to channel energy, all of the assistant instructors sitting cross-legged on either side of her started vibrating with blissful expressions on their faces. All she had to do was focus their minds on orgasmic energy and they started streaming those great juices up and down their bodies.

At the time, this was highly frustrating to me. I was in the midst of weeks of practice before having my first inkling of what they could turn on and off at will. But it sure served as a strong motivator, a reminder of what was possible.

Transformative Powers

Where do you channel the energy you learn to generate through Orgasmic Breathing? Why, up your inner flute, my dear. You may have an overwhelming abundance of energetic juice in your first chakra, your sex center at the base of your spine. You know what happens if you let it simmer and boil. Right, it explodes out the end of vajra. Instead, move the energy up to the belly, the solar plexus, the heart, the brain, and above. Then it excites, enlivens, and enriches your whole body.

Remember my dear friend, Doc Steven, who never chooses explosive orgasms while having multiple inner ones? When I asked him why he never ejaculates, he said, "I just love women so much. When I'm making love, I simply move that juicy orgasmic energy up to my heart. It makes me so high, engulfing me in love. I never want to ejaculate so I can go on merging like that forever." And he really does.

Many ancient texts proclaim the transformative power of moving orgasmic energy even higher, to the throat, brain, third eye behind the eyebrows, and the crown of the head. If you're aiming to raise awareness, it makes total sense to wash the brain with this concentrated life force. More than anything, this is what generates implosive orgasms. When your whole body is vibrating with these waves, you enter the still, empty, timeless void and want to stay there indefinitely.

The tools you know well by now are what you use to create and prolong the experience. In addition to Orgasmic Breathing, you can use peaking, plateauing, and even interrupting ejaculation as needed to keep the flow going. Give feedback, ask yes/no questions, and negotiate different positions as the urge strikes you.

MAKING LOVE ENERGETICALLY

On one end of the sexual spectrum is "Wham, bam, thank you ma'am." On the other end is Orgasmic Energy LovePlay. This blossoms when you take the time and care to create the right environment, mood, setting, and physical space. I call this creating the space for Energy LovePlay. But please realize that the term space means more than just the room you're in.

Exercise: Creating The Space For Energy LovePlay

To enjoy the perfect mood, environment, and space for Energy LovePlay, you need to consciously create the setting, honor each other, connect mentally and emotionally, and open your energy channels, all together. As I've said again and again, entering into Orgasmic Energy LovePlay doesn't work well with a fixed agenda. But I'm going to give you one for your "Creating the Space for Energy LovePlay" Exercise purely as a teaching tool. Once you get the hang of it and discover what gets both your juices going, do it your own way. Here are the directions:

1) Setting: Get everything ready and create the physical space together. Clean the area and pick up books, dirty clothes, and anything extraneous. Get your sound system

and music ready. Collect sacred objects, incense, massage oil, condoms, and lubricant. Decorate the setting with flowers, lighted candles, and beautiful art.

2) Honoring: Welcome each other into the space you've created together with your mind, your eyes, and your words. A wonderful way to begin honoring each other is with a namasté, the traditional Eastern gesture of bowing from the waist with hands on heart, palms together pointing up. To decide together what you both want to do, discuss your desires, concerns (especially regarding sexual practices with a new partner), and boundaries. Be sure to verbally accept your partner's preferences and limits. Exchange gifts, words of love, and gratitude.

3) Connecting: Take a few moments to look deeply into each other's eyes. Ritually undress each other, caressing and complimenting each other's bodies. Share a ritual bath or shower, gently washing the outside world of each other. Merge into a long melting hug with all parts of your bodies touching while synchronizing your breathing.

4) Energizing: Assist each other in opening all your senses. Lightly massage each other's face and hair while whispering sweet everythings (those are the positive version of sweet nothings). Relax each other by slowly massaging your hands and feet with a little oil. Do Orgasmic Breathing together. Lightly caress everywhere on your partner's body, visualizing energy streaming from your heart, down your arms, into your hands, and into your partner's body.

Once you know how to create the space for Energy LovePlay your way, you can move right into the following Shangri-La Exercise at this point. Just remember, there's no way to get it wrong. Listen to your heart, share feelings with your partner, and do what seems right in the moment.

When you don't have all day, you might do an abbreviated version of these things within 10 or 15 minutes. When you really want to go deep and long, spend an hour or more creating the space for Energy LovePlay.

As a typical modern male, I used to resist the ritual aspect of this exercise. Then one day I realized that these preparations made me enter lovemaking in a completely different mood. I learned to drop this resistance so I could open to running energy. So, before dismissing it as useless spiritual hoopla, try it with an open mind and see how it makes you feel.

And face it, guys, women love this kind of syrupy stuff. Remember what the Eagles said on their Hell Freezes Over rock tour after a 14-year breakup? Get over it!

Exercise: Shangri-La

As I remember the story, Shangri-La was some sort of idyllic mountain valley in the Himalayas where everything was beautiful and everyone was happy all the time. Embrace LovePlay as presented here and you'll be transported there. You may not want to leave. And now that you have the skills to make love for hours, you don't have to leave.

Oddly enough, some call this experience of riding the wave of ecstasy the Valley Orgasm. It's not a peak, nor really a plateau. It's more like sinking into an ocean of rapture and letting the current carry you. Maybe I mixed metaphors there, but there's no way words can describe the altered state.

The Shangri-La practice is designed so that you can integrate everything you've learned and realize the vision together. It's about long lovemaking, energy exchange, and maximum ecstasy. Though you may be swept away, explosive orgasm isn't the goal. Multiple inner orgasms are likely, but the purpose of this exercise is creating as much pleasure as you can for as long as you want.

Though it isn't essential, this exercise is best done in the Yab-Yum position, which is the Buddhist name for the union of mother and father. In Yab-Yum, you sit cross-legged, usually on pillows to raise your hips off the floor. Your lover sits on your lap with her legs wrapped around your back. Pillows under her butt and your legs sometimes help.

Alternatively, your partner can squat on your lap with her feet on either side of your hips. In this way she can support her weight and gain more freedom of movement. Or you can use an armless chair. Or both of you can lean back from the Yab-Yum position supporting your weight with your arms stretched out behind you. Experiment to find what's comfortable enough to last for a while.

1) Create the sacred space using the previous exercise.

2) Alternate giving and receiving manual and oral jewel stimulation, moving into sexual union (intercourse) when you both can't wait any longer.

3) Make love slowly and sensuously in various postures until you're both really turned on.

4) Move into the Yab-Yum position or an alternate position that allows your chakras to align next to each other. If you can't get comfortable with your partner on your lap, try spooning or one of you lying on top of the other.

5) Begin slowly rocking your hips together, squeezing your PC pumps and synchronizing your breathing. Visualize the energy moving up your inner flutes as you thrust inside.

6) When you peak on the edge of orgasm, both stop moving, relax completely, but keep breathing together. Visualize the energy of your first chakras, your sex centers at the base of your spine, swirling between you. Use your PC to pump energy upward together.

7) After a few minutes, certainly before you lose your Shiva Lingam, move again until you reach another peak just before the point of no return. This time, exchange energy at the second chakra, just below your navels.

8) Repeat the cycle at each chakra: third at the solar plexus, fourth at the heart, fifth at the throat, sixth at the third eye in the forehead, and the seventh at the crown of the head. You can stroke the front of each other's bodies lightly to encourage your partner's energy to move up.

9) Now continue making love without structure, just letting the surge of energy unfold on its own. Maintain eye contact from time to time and use mouth-to-mouth inverted breathing to heighten your experience. That means you breathe in while your partner breathes out and vice versa. Use your PC pumps to propel the energy up your inner flutes just before exploding. Ride the wave that blossoms within you, wherever it takes you both, without conscious direction.

10) Close together by coming down slowly. Just lie down entwined, or spoon, while your breathing settles. Talk quietly, sharing what you experienced. Conclude with a namasté.

Books have been written about the Shangri-La experience. There's so much variation that moving, breathing, visualizing, and making sounds can bring. Now you've got the tools to be a virtuoso. All you need is creative practice.

CHAPTER 9

✧ *Final Thoughts*

Just as Chapter 1 had an erotic story, so this last chapter begins with a fantasy tale, one based on an actual experience. Imagine yourself in this picture. It could be you on the one-year anniversary of practicing Male Multiple Orgasm, and your future state of ecstasy. It's like watching your own final exam, but one in which all you need to do is read and enjoy. The rest of these final thoughts of the Male Multiple Orgasm mostly contain some vital data about smart sex, and concludes with a discussion of Hands-On Coaching, as well as links to my Web address.

Another Story: This Could Be You

The following fantasy is based on one actual amazing ecstatic evening. Imagine that it's YOU enjoying your one-year anniversary of starting the Male Multiple Orgasm...

Your lover's invitation to join her for dinner and a whole night of play is exciting but cryptic. Her innuendos really turn you on, but you aren't sure what to expect.

As twilight settles, you enter her beautifully decorated temple. You can't help but be titillated by the candlelight, incense, and soft music. You shiver at the way she looks draped sensuously across pillows covering the floor. She's only wearing a little diaphanous fabric. She beckons you to sit next to her and begins feeding you with her fingers. When a morsel "accidentally" slips onto her silky exposed skin, she guides you with a little pout to use your mouth to lick her clean. Giggling together, it's easy to encourage her to eat off of your body, too.

Honoring the God/Goddess Within

After you both have enough finger-food and delightful champagne, she takes your hand and guides you to the bed. You bow, touch foreheads, and look deeply into each other's eyes. One after another, she whispers all the things she loves about your body, mind, and spirit. Similar words of love and affection can't be restrained from gushing out of you.

She slowly begins undressing you, breathing, kissing, and nibbling on each part she so delicately exposes. Accidentally on purpose, she brushes a now-throbbing vajra once or twice. As you return the favor and adore every inch of her body, vajra feels like a rock. Then she leads you into the bath, where you gently wash and dry each other all over.

As she spreads her delightful form on the bed again, she hands you a bottle of scented massage oil. As you touch and caress her sensually, your hands feel the heat from your two hearts meeting. Swooning, you worship every millimeter of her body with sweet oil, slowly and tenderly. When, after another CD changes, you finally touch yoni, she's already dripping with delight. As you delicately play with her sweet flower with your fingers for the longest time, her pleasure streams up your arms, making you feel as if it was your yoni that was being loved.

What's That Juicy Aroma?

All at once, you realize you're face down and she's straddling you. Is that delicious fragrance coating your back the same oil you used, or is it her wet yoni lips? You drop the thought and sink into the juicy massage. Her soft slow touch magnifies the subtle vibrations you're feeling inside into powerful waves of ecstatic spasms.

Suddenly, she rolls you both over and her mouth encircles vajra. Like a tidal wave in an already stormy sea, *a huge surge of energy sweeps up your body, shaking every cell with electric joy. As she sucks, pulse after pulse of pure bliss pumps through you and out the top of your head. On and on she licks and kisses vajra, rocking you inside with liquid fireworks. Floating on some other plane of existence, your mind empties, your body expands to fill the whole room, and your spirit soars in rapture.*

Then a little part of you comes back to earth, realizing your beloved is sitting on you with vajra completely engulfed by yoni, slowly rolling her hips back and forth. As electric fire floods you inside and out, all you can do to contain so much energy is relax completely and breathe. Suddenly, you're floating on that cloud again, but this time together, writhing slowly like snakes intertwined around each other.

Another Place and Time

Some keen other-worldly sense of sight inside you watches as each stroke of vajra propels bolts of lightning through your merged bodies, not two but one huge erogenous zone. After each subtle movement, you float together for minutes, ecstasy streaming out of every pore. Higher and higher the valleys of pleasure rise as you pulse over and over and then surrender to the tide of rapture.

You both lose all sense of time, all sense of physical boundaries, all sense of separation from each other and everything around you. You are one, unified with the universe. Do you need or want anything? No, you're complete. What's next? Nothing, just stay here. Where is that dream life you used to live? Far away.

And then the sun rises.

HAVE LOTS OF SEX— BUT BE SMART AND STAY SAFE

The philosophy of Male Multiple Orgasm says "yes" to whatever you desire with consciousness. I may advocate open sexuality in any form you choose, but not in an unconscious or unsafe manner. Serious STDs (sexually transmitted diseases) such as HIV (the AIDS virus) and hepatitis are believed to be transmitted through fluid exchange. To stay healthy and free from STDs, we all need to be careful and conscious with all sexual contact.

I strongly urge all sexual players and partners to follow the smart sex practices included here. At Tantra At Tahoe, we've adapted the color-coded chart "A Spectrum of the Risks for HIV Transmission" and guidelines from what we learned through the Human Awareness Institute. HAI taught us to play in the green zone and never in the red or pink zones. We suggest the yellow zone is up to individual discretion based on trust and confidence.

A Spectrum of the Risks for HIV Transmission

Red
- ANAL INTERCOURSE without a condom
- Sharing NEEDLES without sterilization
- BLOOD-BLOOD or SEMEN-BLOOD contact

Pink
- ORAL SEX with a man or woman EJACULATING in the mouth
- ORAL SEX with a woman MENSTRUATING
- VAGINAL INTERCOURSE without protection

Yellow
- Sharing SEX TOYS (vibrators, dildos, etc.)
- RIMMING (using the tongue around the anus)
- ORAL SEX on a man without EJACULATING
- ORAL SEX on a woman not MENSTRUATING

Yellow
- URINE in the mouth
- Mutual EROTIC MASSAGE with hands
- FINGERING or FISTING in the vagina or anus
- VAGINAL or ANAL INTERCOURSE with protection

Green
- Simultaneous parallel SELF-PLEASURING
- FROTTAGE (body to body rubbing)
- SOCIAL (dry) KISSING

- FRENCH (wet) KISSING
- PHONE or COMPUTER sex
- VOYEURISM or EXHIBITIONISM
- HOT TUBBING
- HUGGING or MASSAGING

A Smart Sex Conversation

We use the following conversation agenda to be responsible for our own pleasure and decide what level of risk we're comfortable with during each sexual encounter:

I. Desires: Discuss what you want to do.

II. Background: Have a frank, responsible pre-sex conversation:

    1. Brief relevant history of sexual practices

    2. Current sexual practices

        a) high risk

        b) protection

        c) multiple partners

    3. Complete history of STDs

        a) HIV and AIDS

        b) hepatitis

        c) herpes and genital warts

        d) chlamydia, syphilis, and gonorrhea

    4. Most recent STD test results

    5. Skin, mouth, and genital condition

III. Boundaries: Establish and agree on practices and limits.

HANDS-ON COACHING

In spite of the growing interest in Tantra and spiritual sexuality, this vision of sacred lovemaking and intimate communion is rather foreign to many modern Westerners. You can learn much from reading, but as you now know, EXPERIENCE is really where it's at. For this reason, many students new to spiritual sexuality attend workshops and work privately with coaches.

Tantra At Tahoe

Here at Tantra At Tahoe (that's Jeffre and me), we specialize in a series of multi-day **Private Tantra Workshops**, which catapult you quickly into this altered state. By focusing on the needs of one or two people at a time, we can teach practices and rituals that are perfect for unblocking your energy channels and recharging your relationships.

If Tantra is the fast track to enlightenment, our yearlong **Advanced Tantra Initiations** are the customized, super fast track to great lovemaking.

If you want to go deeper, faster into sacred sexuality, we can help customize lessons, long distance training, or home study for you. Please contact us via email here: www.TantraAtTahoe.com/connect/feedback.htm. Or visit our website: www.TantraAtTahoe.com, which describes all of the services mentioned here in greater detail.

By the way, we also conduct Tantra workshops organized by other groups. If you have a circle of close friends, we'd be happy to arrange something for your small group, as well.

Personal Sexuality Coaching

If you're having trouble with the exercises in this book, or you run into other sexual problems, I'm available for Sexuality Coaching. We can do this in person if you are close to Northern California or want to join me during a trip or vacation. Or we can make great progress via telephone or email dialogue. My services are highly professional, totally confidential, and completely respectful of whatever you're experiencing and whatever you desire. Please feel comfortable contacting me with whatever's on your mind here at: somraj@tantraattahoe.com.

✧ *Glossary of Terms*

Any new field that changes human perception and behavior evolves its own lingo. The salient advantage of coining new words is our ability to more precisely focus on ethereal qualities that are difficult to describe with common English. This glossary defines various terms used throughout the book.

9.9   The point of no return, measured on the 10-point scale of sexual arousal at which ejaculatory orgasm is inevitable.

10-Point Scale   An arbitrary way of monitoring level of sexual arousal during practice and sex play from 1, no arousal, to 10, orgasm.

AIDS   Autoimmune Deficiency Syndrome, a disease that destroys the body's ability to fight infections. *See* HIV.

Balls   Slang term for a man's testicles.

Big O   A strong, explosive orgasm.

Chakra   One of seven centers or vortices inside the body, from the bottom of the spine to the top of the head, where subtle energy is generated, collected, stored, and swirled. Though energy is energy, it has different qualities at each chakra. *See* Energy.

Channel Energy   To circulate, move, or run sexual energy around the body. *See* Energy.

Chi   *See* Energy.

Clio   Another name for clitoris. *See* Clitoris.

Clitoris   A female sexual organ above the vagina that can give a woman sexual pleasure when it is touched. *See* Clio.

Coitus Reservatus or **Coitus Interruptus**   The withdrawal technique dating from ancient Rome in which the man pulls his penis out of a woman's vagina before ejaculating.

Come   Slang term for ejaculation.

Cornerstones   Four simple but powerful physical skills used to generate ecstasy at will: presence (relaxation, mental focus, and concentration), breath, sound, and movement.

Corona   The ridge at the base of the head of the penis. Also known as the crown.

Crown   *See* Corona.

Desensitizing   Using products or techniques to temporarily lessen the penis's response during sexual stimulation.

Devamani   A man's scrotum and testicles, adapted from the Sanskrit for divine gems, jewels, or pearls.

Dry Orgasm   A long series of slow, pleasurable spasms that men can experience without ejaculating. *See* Implosive Orgasms.

Ejaculation   To push out semen from the penis, often during orgasm.

Emission Phase   The first stage of ejaculatory orgasm, when the male prostate gland automatically contracts and empties prostatic fluid, a major component of semen, into the urethra.

Energy   The nervous stimulation and physical excitation that our bodies feel all the time. Energy is responsible for emotional sensations and the physical manifestation of spirit. In China, this life force is called chi; in India, it's called prana; and in Japan, it's called ki.

Energy Orgasm   *See* Implosive Orgasm.

Erection   The firm, enlarged state of a man's penis during sexual arousal.

Explosive Orgasm   The kind of sudden, strong orgasm that relieves tension and releases energy quickly in a few-second flash of pleasure, which is accompanied by ejaculation in men.

Expulsion Phase   The rhythmic, wave-like soft muscle contractions that propel semen down a man's urethra and out the head of his penis.

Feedback Sandwich or Feedback Cycle   A communication technique beginning and ending with positive reinforcement, which starts with a compliment, asks for something different, and finally acknowledges what's working. It's a diplomatic way lovers can ask for changes in sexual play or other behavior without hurting a partner's feelings.

Frenulum   The ring of indentation just behind the corona or head of the penis, especially on the underside, which is highly sensitive.

Full Body Orgasm   An energetic implosive orgasm through the entire body, accompanied by writhing, undulating, and vibrating all over as a result of channeling sexual energy. *See* Implosive Orgasm.

Glans   The rounded tip of the clitoris or penis.

G-Spot   A small pleasure point located a few inches deep on the upper part of the vaginal channel, first reported in the 1950s by a gynecologist, Dr. Ernest Grafenberg, as the female orgasmic trigger. Recent research by Dr. Gary Schubach indicates that there actually is a G-area along much of the roof of the vagina along the sponge surrounding the urethra.

Guru   A spiritual teacher or master, traditionally from India.

Hand Job   Manually pleasuring a penis by oneself or by a lover.

Hard-On   A slang term for a male erection.

Head   The glans, corona, or crown of the penis.

HIV   The human immunodeficiency virus that causes AIDS, a disease that destroys the body's ability to fight infections.

Implosive Orgasm   A long series of slow, pleasurable vibrations in both men and women, accompanied by a rush of orgasmic energy. Men can experience an implosive orgasm without ejaculating. Also called inner orgasm or energy orgasm. *See* Dry Orgasm.

Imsak   An Arabic word literally meaning "retention"—referring to retaining semen within the body while making love. Imsak was developed for men who needed to satisfy an entire harem each night and couldn't keep getting it up again and again.

Inner Flute   The invisible channel, imagined to look like a hollow bamboo, near the spine that connects the chakras. *See* Chakra.

Jewels   A Tantric term for both male and female sex organs.

Karezza   A lovemaking technique in which the penis remains motionless inside the vagina for an hour or more, simply feeling the delightful energy. First published by Alice Bunker Stockham, a pioneering female physician, in 1883.

Kegels   Exercises that help women restore muscle tone and regain control of their urinary reflexes after the trauma of childbirth. Kegels were originally developed in 1952 by a gynecologist named Dr. Arnold Kegel. *See* PC Muscle.

Ki   *See* Energy.

Lingam   The Hindu name for penis. *See* Vajra.

Lotus Position   Sitting with knees bent and legs crossed over one another.

Meditation   A technique to empty and clear the mind by reciting mantras, watching the breath, or witnessing ideas floating by. Meditation is intended to create a "no mind" condition of deep inner peace filled with stillness.

Move Energy   To circulate, channel, or run sexual energy around the body. *See* Energy.

Namasté   Bowing from the waist with hands on heart, palms together pointing up, meaning "the God/Goddess within me salutes the God/Goddess within you."

No Mind   A meditative state of deep inner peace filled with stillness.

Orgasm   Sexual climax, the moment of most intense pleasure in sexual stimulation, usually accompanied with explosive release, and sometimes by an unlimited, timeless, whole body-mind-spirit altered state.

Orgasm Master   Someone who can choose the type, timing, and number of orgasms that occur.

Orgasmic Energy   *See* Energy.

PC Muscle   Short for pubococcygeus. The muscle that snakes down around the anus and jewels connecting the pubic to the coccyx bones plus the sitting bones and legs.

Peak   Letting sexual excitement rise to a high level and then immediately drop back down, which, if graphed, looks like scaling a steep mountain peak and then falling precipitously.

Peaking   Adjusting the sexual stimuli that cause sudden surges of arousal in order to come back down without going over the top to orgasm.

Performance Anxiety   The worry of a lover who's trying to achieve a goal like orgasm, competing with internal mental standards, and continuously wondering, "Am I doing it right?"

Perineum   The general region of the pelvic floor between the jewels and rosetta (anus).

PIV   Penis in vagina.

Plateau An ongoing high level of sexual arousal that continues without diminishing.

PNV Penis near vagina.

Point of No Return The moment during sexual arousal at which ejaculatory orgasm is inevitable. *See* 9.9.

Polyamory An open lifestyle that includes multiple lovers.

Prana *See* Energy.

Prostate A firm, partly muscular, chestnut-sized gland located a long finger-width inside the rectum of males at the neck of the urethra. It produces prostatic fluid, a viscous secretion that is a primary component of semen.

Prostate Point A soft spot between the devamani (testicles) and rosetta (anus), below the base of the penis, through which pressure can be applied to the prostate.

Prostatitis An inflamed or enlarged prostate.

RAMPER The best method of teaching the Male Multiple Orgasm. RAMPER stands for: **R**elax, **A**wareness, **M**easure, **P**ace, **E**nergy circulation, and **R**ide the wave.

Refractory Period The time it takes to be able to recover the ability to get and maintain an erection after ejaculating.

Retention Conserving or retaining semen without ejaculating during sex.

Rosetta Anus.

Run Energy To circulate, channel, or move sexual energy around the body. *See* Energy.

Sacred Spot *See* G-Spot.

Scrotum The external pouch hanging behind a man's penis that contains the testicles.

Self-Pleasuring Preferred term for masturbation during which one honors one's body and celebrates pleasure.

Semen   Seed, seminal fluid, or ejaculate. The thick white fluid containing spermatozoa that is ejaculated by the male during sexual release.

Sensate focus   Tuning in to all your senses: taste, touch, sight, sound, and smell. It means delighting in every sight, basking in every fragrance, and savoring every sensation.

S.E.X.   Subtle Energy eXchange. Any touching, moving, meditating, or erotic sharing, including fantasy, that stimulates and connects lovers' inner vibrations.

Sexual Energy   *See* Energy.

Shakti   The goddess, Shiva's consort, that represents the feminine principle embodying pure creative energy.

Shiva   The god Shiva, one of the three primary Hindu deities, known in Tantra as the pure embodiment of masculine force and cosmic consciousness.

Shiva Lingam   An erect penis. Tantric tradition views the all-powerful God Shiva with a continuous erection.

Signals   Words, sounds, or hand motions used to give feedback to a sexual partner about erotic reactions and arousal level.

Sperm   Spermatozoa, the male reproductive cells.

STD   Sexually transmitted disease.

Streaming   To circulate, move, run, or channel sexual energy, often without sexual stimulation, which creates strong pleasurable spasms and vibrations.

Taking Touch   A massage technique where the touching hand feels as much as the body part that's being caressed.

Tantra   The ancient spiritual science of sacred sex.

Tantras   Ancient secret writings about Tantra.

Tantrikas   Practitioners adept at Tantra.

Urethra   The tube or canal through which urine is discharged in both men and women. The urethra also serves as the male genital duct that carries semen through the genital system and out the head of the penis.

Urge to Ejaculate   When a man becomes sexually aroused and a feeling inside takes over and convinces him to just let go.

Vajra   The penis or male sexual organ. *See* Lingam.

Valley Orgasm   A continuous state of orgasmic ecstasy in which the arousal curve stays flat like a mesa and doesn't jump up suddenly, as in peaking. *See* Plateau.

Vipassana Meditation   A sensory meditation designed to open multiple senses at once.

VIY   Vajra In Yoni.

VNY   Vajra Near Yoni.

Yab-Yum   The paramount sexual position named for the Buddhist term "union of mother and father"—in which the man sits cross-legged with the woman on his lap with her legs wrapped around him.

Yang   Strong male energy.

Yes/No Questions   One-word questions, can be answered with a simple "yes" or "no," allowing lovers to give feedback without thinking much.

Yin   Receptive female energy.

Yoni   The traditional Hindu word for a woman's vagina.

Zafu   A solid, round Japanese meditation pillow, flattened top and bottom like a thick pancake.

✧ *Resources*

BOOK RECOMMENDATIONS

Tantra At Tahoe Books

Go to http://www.TantraAtTahoe.com/product/books.htm for detailed information and immediate download of our growing Tantric Sex Book Library...

Supreme Bliss Tantra

Our Tantra beginners guidebook is a rich, easy-to-follow, how-to guide that teaches the joys of Spiritual Sex so you can merge sex and spirit, make loveplay sacred, deepen your love and connection, and unleash your dormant passion to soar in awesome ecstasy. Though it's for Tantra beginners, many of the 101 exercises in our richly illustrated lovemaking manual are great for lovers of all ages.

Tantric G-Spot Orgasm & Female Ejaculation: Awakening Her Sacred Gate To Supreme Bliss

Here's the complete guidebook to supercharging your sexual play with Female Ejaculation and Tantric G-Spot Orgasms of incredible power and emotional sweetness. No longer will your or your lover's G-Spot be mysterious and elusive. Read our book to know exactly how to awaken it, find it, and touch it for supreme pleasure. With frank language, step-by-step instructions, real pictures, and clear charts, you'll learn how to excite the G-Spot with fingers, tongues, and sexual intercourse. Our new how-to sex manual guides you to expand your capacity for pleasure by giving and receiving the amazing ecstasy of Female Ejaculation.

Tantric Male: Multiple G-Spot Orgasm

Men, learn to awaken your secret orgasmic trigger. Women, become every man's dream lover by learning how to give unlimited male multiple orgasms with our book about giving and receiving the ecstatic pleasure of male prostate massage. It's chock full of frank, accurate, detailed, up-to-date information and 49 graphic color photos and charts about male sexual anatomy. Our male G-Spot book includes 47 exciting solo and hands-on partner practices that will show you exactly how to find, excite, and create incredible pleasure from your own or your partner's G-Spot.

Intimacy, A Green Light For Red Hot Sex
And A Lifetime Of Loving

The fuel for an enduring, sexy, passionate, love affair is an ever-growing depth of intimacy, which opens the door to an ever-evolving red hot sex life. Our practical, exciting relationship book shows you step-by-step how to use romance and flirting to juice up your sex life while sweetening your relationship. Jeffre's sizzling playbook gives you the lovemaking tools, Tantric sex tips, and sex education to make your sexual relationship hotter than ever.

Books for Further Study

The Art Of Sexual Ecstasy: The Path Of Sacred Sexuality For Western Lovers by Margo Anand, Jeremy P. Tarcher, Los Angeles, 1989

What can I say, this is our teacher's book, the book that started us on the ecstatic Tantric path. It's the most comprehensive practical system, replete with exercises and practices that you'll want to pore over and do again and again.

The Art Of Sexual Magic: Cultivating Sexual Energy To Transform Your Life by Margo Anand, Jeremy P. Tarcher, Los Angeles, 1995

An advanced course in erotic enchantment and the magic of extended orgasm, which takes the power of sexuality beyond mere lovemaking by showing readers how to generate intense sexual energy and use it as fuel for realizing personal and spiritual goals.

Divine Sex: The Tantric & Taoist Arts Of Conscious Loving by Caroline Aldred, HarperSanFrancisco, 1996

A beautiful, short, glossy illustrated paperback that summarizes the sacred approach to lovemaking.

ESO: How You And Your Lover Can Give Each Other Hours Of Extended Sexual Orgasm by Alan P. Brauer, M.D., and Donna J. Brauer, Warner Books, New York, 1983

This is a short but groundbreaking book with a workable method for separating ejaculation from orgasm and extending loveplay. It really makes clear how much sexual potential the average lover never activates. Though somewhat clinical and non-spiritual, as you'd expect from a physician, it gives physical exercises to make both men's and women's orgasms reach inconceivable new heights and go on forever.

How To Make Love All Night (and Drive A Woman Wild): Male Multiple Orgasm And Other Secrets For Prolonged Lovemaking by Barbara Keesling, Ph.D., HarperPerrenial, New York, 1994

A short, pragmatic paperback by a female psychologist who explains exactly how she teaches clients to do what her title promises.

The Love Keys: The Art Of Ecstatic Sex by Diana Richardson, Harper Collins, UK, 1999

This may be my favorite Tantric book of all time. It's a perfect blend of the Tantric weaving of heart, spirit, lust, ritual and practicality. Diana is quite opinionated about many unique practices, which all bear experimentation.

The New Male Sexuality: The Truth About Men, Sex, And Pleasure by Bernie Zilbergeld, Ph.D., Bantam Books, New York, 1992

This is the top scientific book by one of the leading sex therapists about male sexuality, complete with frank discussion of all benefits and problems, including many practical exercises.

The One Hour Orgasm: The Ultimate Guide To Totally Satisfying Any Man Or Woman Every Time! by Dr. Bob Schwartz, Ph.D. and Leah Schwartz, Breakthrough Publishing, Houston, 1995

This book contains great exercises to deliver on its flagrant promise. It's based on 25 years of research by More University, which teaches sensuality and erotic practice, focused primarily on how to satisfy women.

Sacred Sex: Ecstatic Techniques for Empowering Relationships by Jwala (Kathleen Bingham), Inner Juice Productions, San Francisco, 1993

A beautiful little book that teaches a 3-hour Tantric ritual, including many unique and powerful exercises for individual preparation and couple bonding.

Sexual Energy Ecstasy: A Practical Guide To Lovemaking Secrets Of The East And West by David and Ellen Ramsdale, Bantam Books, New York, 1985

The most practical and technique-filled book about creating and maximizing the ecstatic response during lovemaking. Very spiritual and, as you might expect from the title, focused on maximizing sexual energy.

Sexual Secrets: The Alchemy of Ecstasy by Nik Douglas and Penny Slinger, Destiny Books, Rochester, Vermont, 1979

This is an amazing compilation of practices and rituals from ancient texts in language and graphics useful to the modern

Tantrika. Nik and Penny have done a great service to the modern world by giving us access to these hidden secrets.

Spiritual Sex: Secrets Of Tantra From The Ice Age To The New Millennium by Nik Douglas, Pocket Books, New York, 1997

A thorough review of the history of Tantra and sacred sexuality, including a concise summary of modern Tantric practice.

Sexual Solutions: A Guide For Men And The Women Who Love Them by Michael Castleman, Touchstone, New York, 1980

This is a down-to-earth, no nonsense, review of male sexual problems and techniques to improve lovemaking. A little dry and devoid of spirit for me, but worthwhile for its helpful exercises.

Tantra: The Art Of Conscious Loving by Charles & Caroline Muir, Mercury House, San Francisco, 1989

A wonderful little book that presents the Muirs' approach to teaching Tantra, weaving Yoga, relationship, and sexual healing into erotic practice.

Taoist Secrets Of Love: Cultivating Male Sexual Energy by Mantak Chia and Michael Winn, Aurora Press, Santa Fe, New Mexico, 1984

This is an excellent presentation of the Taoist approach to male sexuality, which prescribes and is apparently successful in achieving complete seminal retention for men. It has some powerful exercises, but is too strict and preachy for Tantrikas like me.

The Three-Week Program Ending Premature Ejaculation: Man's Guide To Self-Improvement To Help Improve Sensual Awareness by William L. Nakosan, Minimum W. Publishers, New York, 1994

This is an English translation of *The Simple Solution*, a short little paperback basically presenting a frank discussion of the situation and exercises to practice coming close and backing off.

The Yin-Yang Butterfly: Ancient Chinese Sexual Secrets For Western Lovers by Valentin Chin, Jeremy P. Tarcher/Putnam, New York, 1994

A decidedly Taoist version of ancient sexual secrets, which is more regimented than much Tantric practice, but contains some valuable tools and rituals.

MUSIC RECOMMENDATIONS

Tantric Practice Music

El-Hadra: the Mystik Dance by Klaus Wiese, Ted de Jong, Mathia Grassow

The rhythm of Sufi trance meditation. One of our key practice CDs that we use to teach Orgasmic Breathing and moving energy up your chakras. This rhythmic, moving background piece was specially produced for our teacher, Margot Anand. Just listening to it makes us stream sexual energy.

Dorje Ling by David Parsons

A slow, rhythmic, moving mix that samples traditional Tibetan music with a gently evolving electronic composition. The first 14-minute track is called "Tantra."

Passion by Peter Gabriel

Over 20 short tracks with mostly subtle rhythms, composed as the score for the "Last Temptation of Christ." Often melodic and sensuous, sometimes quiet, sometimes raucous with a Middle Eastern flair.

Deep Forest, Boheme, and *Comparsa* by Deep Forest

I don't know if these guys really are African or are Western New Age musicians playing earthy sounds. Regardless, the primal nature of Deep Forest's music is great for dancing, moving the hips, and getting sexual energy flowing.

Totem and Bones by Gabrielle Roth and the Mirrors

Jeffre loves drums and primitive rhythms so Gabrielle's simple beat turns her on more than most, who simply find them trance-like.

Relaxing Meditative Music

SAN by Deuter

The consummate New Age musician who's responsible for the dynamic music on many of our meditation CDs uses his gentle touch for this series of soft, subtle, relaxing themes.

Tantric Heart: Music For Lovers by Shastro

Two long, slow, sensual tracks inspired by Indian themes, which are energizing and relaxing.

Higher Ground and Sensual Pleasure plus others by Steven Halpern

Evocative, sustained chords float, suspended in time, amply meditative and relaxing.

Tantra Drums by Al Gromer Khan

Mystical, flowing, sensual, erotic, engaging... lovely musical support for slow, ecstatic lovemaking. Transports the listener to another level of consciousness.

Music To Disappear In 1 & 2 by Raphael

Key elements in the trancey section of our music collection, bound to lull anyone into a timeless space.

Sensual Lovemaking Music

ERA by ERA

The eerie chanting and vocals of ERA are hip and upbeat, creating an erotic mood.

Erotic Moods by Nusound

A rhythmic, sensual, romantic musical journey punctuated by lush electronic sounds.

Mythos by Mythos

This upbeat group centered on piano and guitar—but with many other instruments in places—is our latest favorite, featuring a timeless feeling of mysticism through African, Middle Eastern, and Oriental tones.

Karma, Poem, Chimera, and *Semantic Spaces* by Delerium

Maybe because we both love rock and roll so much, Delerium has long been one of our top artists for lovemaking. Their three latest CDs put us into an altered space with electronic sound, hypnotic rhythm, and sensual themes. "Poem" has more strong vocals than the earlier two, which pulse right into our subconscious energy centers.

B-Tribe V, Spiritual Spiritual, Sensual Sensual, and *Suave Suave* by B-Tribe

Two of our favorite erotic CDs have some Spanish vocalizing over rock-type flamenco music. Since we don't speak the language, it transports us to a romantic space without thinking.

Enigma, The Cross Of Changes, Le Roi Est Mort, and *The Screen Behind The Mirror* by Enigma

Any new collection of sensual music has to include Enigma's four great CDs. They're a little verbal and changeable, so they don't have the trance-like effect we prefer, but the rich themes and instrumentation make them a joy to listen to.

✧ *Other Books from Amorata Press*

The Best Sex Positions Ever!

Alex Williams, $16.95

Presents an inspirational approach to lovemaking, one designed to take readers to higher peaks of ecstasy through new and stimulating erotic moves.

The Best Sex You'll Ever Have!

Richard Emerson, $13.95

Packed with a variety of new ideas to spice up lovemaking, *The Best Sex You'll Ever Have!* illustrates risque positions, fantasies, role playing, sex toys and erotic games.

The Little Bit Naughty Book of Sex

Dr. Jean Rogiere, $9.95

A handy pocket hardcover that is a fun, full-on guide to enjoying great sex.

The Little Bit Naughty Book of Sex Positions

Siobhan Kelly, $9.95

Fully illustrated with 50 tastefully explicit color photos, *The Little Bit Naughty Book of Sex Positions* provides everything readers need to start using these thrilling new positions tonight.

Naughty Tricks and Sexy Tips: A Couple's Guide to Uninhibited Erotic Pleasure

2nd Edition, Pam Spurr, $10.00

Designed to present quick and easy advice, this book shows couples how to start improving their sex life immediately. It serves up hundreds of bite-sized tidbits that are sure to enhance and expand anyone's sexual repertoire.

Orgasms: A Sensual Guide to Female Ecstasy
Nicci Talbot, $16.95

Straight-talking and informative, *Orgasms* is a girl's best friend when it comes to understanding the physical, psychological, and spiritual factors contributing to great sex and intense orgasms.

Orgasm Every Day Every Way Every Time: A Woman's Guide to Sexual Pleasure
Jenny Wood, $12.95

Dishes up everything from fantastic foreplay tips and mind-blowing masturbation techniques to orgasm-inducing intercourse positions and creative new ways to reach that peak of ecstasy.

Unleashing Her G-Spot Orgasm: A Step-by-Step Guide to Giving a Woman Ultimate Sexual Ecstasy
Donald L. Hicks, $12.95

Drawing on the latest findings of world-renowned sex researchers, this useful handbook offers a unique combination of clinical fact and everyday application.

The Wild Guide to Sex and Loving
Siobhan Kelly, $16.95

Packed with practical, frank and sometimes downright dirty tips on how to hone your bedroom skills, this handbook tells you everything you need to know to unlock the secrets of truly tantalizing sensual play.

To order these books call 800-377-2542 or 510-601-8301, fax 510-601-8307, e-mail ulysses@ulyssespress.com, or write to Ulysses Press, P.O. Box 3440, Berkeley, CA 94703. All retail orders are shipped free of charge. California residents must include sales tax. Allow two to three weeks for delivery.

✧ *About the Author*

Somraj Pokras is the author of 3 business books, 4 Tantra ebooks, and 4 Tantric Sex ecourses, as well as the leader of 50 people skills workshops. As co-founder of TantraAtTahoe.com, he's written hundreds of informative web pages and how-to articles as part of publishing their free weekly newsletter. During his 35-year career as a counselor, group facilitator, and trainer, Somraj has guided more that 20,000 people to lead more effective lives. He derives great joy from assisting others to release inhibitions that block their pleasure so they can enjoy life, love, and ecstatic lovemaking for hours and hours.

Somraj is a private pilot, avid skier, mountain bike rider, website designer, and worshipper of the Goddess. He lives in Truckee, California, in the natural paradise of the Sierra Nevada Mountains near Lake Tahoe, with his beautiful and accomplished Tantric wife and his fun-loving golden retrievers.

TantraAtTahoe.com specializes in Spiritual Sex and Sacred Sexuality ebooks, ecourses, personal coaching, and hands-on training to help lovers create Supreme Bliss. They serve couples and singles seeking to lengthen their lovemaking, deepen their intimacy, and supercharge their orgasms by combining ancient Eastern tools with modern sex research.

Please contact Somraj at TantraAtTahoe.com if you're interested in personal coaching, counseling therapy, private training, or relationship workshops.